MW00465501

Praise for *Learning to Love Midlife*
by Chip Conley

"For many of us, midlife can be a confusing stage of life, full of unfamiliar transitions and few clear milestones. And now that we're living longer, this period lasts much longer than it did in the past. *Learning to Love Midlife* is an invaluable guide to how to navigate this period with curiosity, energy, and optimism. With cutting-edge research, deep insight, and examples drawn from real life—including candid accounts of his own experience— Conley provides a clear blueprint for creating the lives we want."

—Gretchen Rubin, bestselling author of
The Happiness Project and *Life in Five Senses*

"I've personally experienced the magic of midlife at Chip Conley's MEA, where thousands of people have learned how to curate a life that's as deep and meaningful as it is long. Finally, Chip has gathered the secrets of that program into a book that will help you to feel happier, healthier, and wiser starting in your 40s."

—Dan Buettner, *New York Times* bestselling
author, creator of "The Blue Zones," and
National Geographic Fellow

"One of the most fascinating developments of this cathartic time we inhabit, surely, is the evolution of aging itself. Chip Conley's work in nourishing and reinventing eldering has been groundbreaking. Now this book is a beautiful offering— spiritual and pragmatic at once— to us all on the generative possibilities of the new midlife. What a joy and a gift it is to read, and to have as a companion for living."

—Krista Tippett, founder and
host of the On Being Project

"As the founder of the world's first midlife wisdom school (I'm an enthusiastic alum!), Chip addresses head-on the question 'What's next?' With his perfect mix of personal anecdotes, professional observation, and social science research, this book is packed with insights to live your life's next best chapter." —Sara Blakely, founder of Spanx

"Chip Conley is a builder. He's a master of making people feel welcome and comfortable even in places where they sometimes fear to tread. Like his legendary retreats, *Learning to Love Midlife* is a warm, hospitable gathering place where readers can learn to embrace their messy selves and transform their lives for the better."

—Bruce Feiler, *New York Times* bestselling author
of *Life Is in the Transitions* and *The Search*

"Does aging give you a sense of dread? If so, you need to read *Learning to Love Midlife* right now. In this wonderful book, Chip Conley will show you that aging is a superpower, capable of changing you (and our world) for the better."

—Arthur C. Brooks, professor, Harvard Kennedy
School and Harvard Business School,
and #1 *New York Times* bestselling
author of *From Strength to Strength*

LEARNING *to*
LOVE
MIDLIFE

ALSO BY CHIP CONLEY

A Year of Wisdom with Chip Conley

Wisdom at Work: The Making of a Modern Elder

*Emotional Equations: Simple Steps for
Creating Happiness + Success in Business + Life*

PEAK: How Great Companies Get Their Mojo from Maslow

*Marketing That Matters: 10 Practices to Profit Your Business
and Change the World*

The Rebel Rules: Daring to Be Yourself in Business

LEARNING *to* LOVE MIDLIFE

12 REASONS WHY LIFE GETS BETTER WITH AGE

CHIP CONLEY

LITTLE, BROWN SPARK

New York Boston London

Little, Brown Spark
Hachette Book Group
1290 Avenue of the Americas, New York, NY 10104
littlebrownspark.com

First Edition: January 2024

Little, Brown Spark is an imprint of Little, Brown and Company, a division of Hachette Book Group, Inc. The Little, Brown Spark name and logo are trademarks of Hachette Book Group, Inc.

The publisher is not responsible for websites (or their content) that are not owned by the publisher.

The Hachette Speakers Bureau provides a wide range of authors for speaking events. To find out more, go to hachettespeakersbureau.com or email HachetteSpeakers@hbgusa.com.

Little, Brown and Company books may be purchased in bulk for business, educational, or promotional use. For information, please contact your local bookseller or the Hachette Book Group Special Markets Department at special.markets@hbgusa.com.

ISBN 9780316567022

An LCCN for this book is available from the Library of Congress

Printing 1, 2023

LSC-C

Printed in the United States of America

*To my two MEA cofounders, Christine Sperber and
Jeff Hamaoui.
The life lessons in this book wouldn't exist without you.*

Contents

Contents

THE VOCATIONAL LIFE

THE SPIRITUAL LIFE

LEARNING *to* LOVE MIDLIFE

Introduction:
A Tale of Two Midlifes

Midlife is the Rodney Dangerfield of life stages: It don't get no respect.

I stared at my ceiling, sleepless in San Francisco, knowing that I would have to fight my battles all over again tomorrow, even more exhausted.

"What's wrong with me?!" That was the question that haunted me in my mid-40s. I hated my life, partly because every piece of it was falling apart. Yet I clung to those pieces as if they were a tattered life preserver.

Worse still, I felt completely alone. An idiot without a village.

Midlife is when we begin to worry that life isn't turning out the way we expected. We may feel a sense of lost opportunity and frustrated longing. Or feel that we've sold out and are living someone else's life. It's when we can look in the mirror and see a stranger.

But once we settle into the transformative opportunity of

3

midlife, something profound and beautiful awakens inside us. For me, this life stage has been the tale of two midlifes: one very bad followed by one very good. Life does get better with age.

I deeply believe that society doesn't understand the upside of this era. We've come to think—and accept—the notion that midlife is one endless sand trap on the golf course of life. Pop culture's most common stereotype about midlife is that our only option is to imitate Kevin Spacey in *American Beauty*: Buy a red 1970 Pontiac Firebird and lust after your teenage daughter's seductive best friend. I know, not a great look!

In short, midlife has a colossal branding problem.

The English word *midlife* dates back to 1818, but it didn't enter the pop-culture lexicon till the mid-1960s. And it was less of a state of life than a trait. Yes, there were twentieth-century midlife markers—menopause, empty nest, parents passing away, twenty-fifth anniversary at work—but to be experiencing midlife was also thought to mean feeling stuck, bored, and dissatisfied. Hence, it was seen almost as an afflic-tion...and a lousy excuse for crazy, selfish behavior.

Is any other era of life yoked so consistently with the term *crisis*, defined as "a time of intense difficulty, trouble, or dan-ger"? Sounds rotten, right? Interestingly, however, the word *crisis* is derived from the Greek word *krinein*, which means "to make a decision based upon one's judgment." In other words, we have agency in our lives. This sheds a different light on the midlife brand, doesn't it? Maybe midlife is not something that happens *to* you, but a life stage that happens *for* you, one that unlocks a whole new world of choices. Wow, that just wiped my windshield clean!

Yale's Dr. Becca Levy has shown that when we shift our perspective on aging from negative to positive, our health outcomes improve. Better balance, more openness to new experiences, better cognitive functioning, more satisfying sex life, and all kinds of other benefits.

She's also shown that we're granted seven and a half years of additional life when we reframe our mindset on aging. Remarkably, this is more additional longevity than if we stop smoking or start exercising at age 50. Where are the public service announcements (PSAs) on the health benefits of reframing aging?!?

This book is meant to be your midlife PSA: a wake-up call (appropriate from a former hotelier, right?) to the unexpected pleasures and joys of midlife. On average, we're becoming wiser, less reactive, more generous, and happier as we get older. Our life has gained a rich patina.

I know this may sound blasphemous in our ageist society, but aging can be far more aspirational than most people realize. Instead of an era one has to endure, midlife can be a time to adore. In the pages ahead, you'll learn why.

Your Midlife Chrysalis

So when do you hit midlife? I know it crept up on me like a lurker in a back alley.

Midlife is generally defined as the years 40 to 65. A growing number of social scientists believe midlife has grown longer recently, as many young knowledge workers feel obsolete earlier due to artificial intelligence and many of us are staying in the workplace longer by choice or necessity. The most conclusive study ever done on midlife development in the United States (*Midlife in the United States*, or MIDUS) studied people 25 to 74 years old.

In my opinion (and that of a growing number of sociologists), in a world with more and more centenarians, midlife may last from 35 to 75. Just as adolescence is a transitional stage between childhood and adulthood, maybe part of midlife's role is to be a transitional stage between adulthood and elderhood.

I believe there are three stages of midlife. During early midlife (years 35 to 50), we tend to experience some of the challenging physical and emotional transitions—a bit like an adult puberty. We realize we are no longer young, but not yet old, and we can feel it's time to metaphorically shed our skin. The core of midlife is our 50s, when we've settled into this new era and are seeing some of the upside—which you'll read about later in this book. Later midlife, which might last from 60 to 75, is when we're young enough to still be working and living a very vital life, but old enough to see and plan for what's next: our senior years. At 63, I am just getting acquainted with this third stage, but I do know it's also when our body reminds us it doesn't want to be forgotten.

Of course, not everyone experiences these three stages on

the same timeline. Midlife is less of an age than it is a feeling. And just as with any other stage of life, *your mileage may vary.*

Taffy Brodesser-Akner is someone whose mileage definitely varied. She is the author of the midlife book and TV series *Fleishman Is in Trouble* and says her midlife crisis happened earlier than most. As Taffy told NPR's *Fresh Air*, at 33, with a one-year-old baby in tow, she wasn't experiencing the wild, professional success she'd imagined for herself: the success her other classmates from film school appeared to enjoy. She says, "The start of middle age hit me like a truck."

On the other hand, my dear old dad, Steve, says his midlife lasted through his mid-70s when he started winding down his career.

Regardless of what age defines it, for many of us, life begins at 50. Before that, life is just a dress rehearsal.

Fortunately, a more life-affirming description of midlife can be found in the dictionary. Go to the Cs, and you'll find *chrysalis,* defined as "a transitional state." When a caterpillar is fully grown, it uses a button of silk to fasten its body to a twig and then forms a chrysalis. Within this protective chrysalis, the transformational magic of metamorphosis occurs. While it's a bit dark, gooey, and solitary, it's a transition, not a crisis. And, of course, on the other side is a beautiful, winged butterfly.

If you yield to the chrysalis call, it means that the incessant accumulating (the caterpillar consuming) must come to an end. This means dropping mindsets, habits, identities, stories, and choices made when we were younger, which no longer reflect who we are or who we're meant to be. As David

Bowie is reported to have said before he passed away, way too young, "Aging is an extraordinary process whereby you become the person you always should have been."

This is a rich time for introspection, a journey through stillness into freedom. We must transcend the caterpillar if our midlife calling is "to butterfly."

A caterpillar consumes. A chrysalis transforms. A butterfly pollinates. Early midlife is when much of what we accumulated dissolves, just before we're ready to transform and pollinate our wisdom to the world in our 50s and beyond.

The Midlife Unraveling

Midlife is the initiation into a time of massive transitions. A drizzle of disappointments. Parents passing away, kids leaving home, financial reckonings, changing jobs, changing spouses, hormonal wackiness, scary health diagnoses, addictive behaviors becoming unwieldy, and the stirring of a growing curiosity about the meaning of life. Author Brené Brown calls this era the "midlife unraveling."

Let's unravel this word *unravel*. My initial reaction to hearing the word was, "Geez, I don't want that to happen to me!" It sounds like something is falling apart.

The more I thought about it, though, the more the word made sense. I experienced that unraveling, as well as a large dose of anxiety, in my mid-to-late 40s. I felt that I had less time to "correct" my life than I had a decade earlier.

Between 45 and 50, I felt like a failure on so many levels. My long-term relationship was ending. My company was falling apart due to the Great Recession. My adult foster son was going to prison for a crime he was wrongfully accused of committing.

It was also a time when I came face-to-face with mortality. I was losing friends and my health was failing. My life was one big unraveling.

"Slightly wounded and tightly wound" was how I described myself to a longtime friend just a couple of weeks before I had my NDE (Near Death Experience) at age 47. My self-esteem was so raveled up and tangled with the way others perceived me that I felt like the hunchback of San Francisco, and not just in my physical body.

For many, midlife can feel like a run-on sentence without any punctuation. It can be a time of deep disappointment in oneself and the world. This might be part of the reason I lost five male midlife friends—most in their 40s—to suicide, right when I was going through my own midlife challenges.

One of them, Chip Hankins, was my mirror. Not only did we share the same preppy nickname, but we were born the same year and were publicly extroverted but had an introverted, melancholy side. Our friends felt comfortable taking quiet counsel with us, and, in fact, Chip was a bit of a spiritual adviser for me.

However, though he was often helping his friends, he didn't admit to himself that he, too, was in a dark tunnel of his own mind's making, silently experiencing deep emotional and physical pain.

Hearing "Chip stories" at Chip's memorial service was surreal. His friends weren't talking about me, but I felt hyper-conscious that I might be the next one to join this private club of those who checked out from life way too early.

It was then that I started telling friends about my night-mares of cancer and car crashes. I felt trapped by the momentum and monotony of my life and was looking for an escape. I was yearning for a midlife pit stop, an off-ramp from an endless freeway where I felt I was running on fumes.

Less than two months after Chip's memorial service, I experienced a miracle disguised as a crisis, a severe allergic reaction to an antibiotic I was taking for a broken ankle and septic leg. I died multiple times onstage just after giving a speech in St. Louis.

My NDE helped me to see how silently unmoored I was from what brought me joy, which was psychologically awkward for a guy who'd started a company named Joie de Vivre (joy of life). My wise, thoughtful friend Bruce Feiler calls the wreck of my world a "lifequake." (Excuse my French, but I called it a clusterfuck. Sorry for swearing, Mom!)

But after experiencing the dark side of early midlife, I found myself in the light around age 50. Within two years of my NDE, I'd sold my company at the bottom of the market, ended my problematic romantic partnership, gotten my foster son exonerated and freed from prison, and realized that my own suicidal ideation was based on the prison of my own constricting identities. And while it wasn't easy, I was able to move on from a career that had defined my identity for two dozen years: being founder and CEO of my boutique hotel company.

With newfound time affluence, I hung out in my backyard hammock listening to Rickie Lee Jones and studying a series of topics that had always fascinated me: the nature of emotions, the growing popularity of festivals, the geophysics that create hot springs.

I got in the best shape of my life, partly because I was in dating mode again. But I also started wondering whether I was irrelevant in the working world. In the film *The Intern*, Robert De Niro says, "Musicians don't retire. They stop when there's no more music in them." I knew I had some "music" to share, but I wasn't sure with whom to share it.

It was around that time, at 52, that I got a call from the cofounder and CEO of a fledgling, fast-growing tech start-up named Airbnb. Brian Chesky asked me if I wanted to help him and his cofounders "democratize hospitality." I initially thought home sharing was a terrible idea. Boy, was I wrong! I wasn't the only hotelier who didn't see this Millennial disruptor sneaking up on us.

I decided to come on board as Brian's in-house mentor and a senior leader, and more than seven years later, Airbnb had grown into the world's most valuable hospitality company, and I was crowned its "modern elder" because they said I was as curious as I was wise. Thank you very much, but less than a decade earlier I'd felt like a "modern failure."

After my challenging transition into midlife in my 40s, I found my 50s to be a revelation. A time when I developed into the man I was always meant to be. It wasn't a perfect decade, but it was a time when I joyfully shed so many of my identities that were no longer serving me. I felt like I was being birthed into a second adulthood.

It was also when my curiosity once again led me to the newest topic I wanted to explore: one of the three life stages that was born in the twentieth century. But, unlike the other two—adolescence and retirement—midlife felt unloved and unstudied. And, when it was studied, it was mostly men studying men. Midlife was a life stage constrained with a bad brand—"midlife crisis"—a term that had been around almost as many years as I had.

Brené says,

> The midlife unraveling is a series of painful nudges strung together by low-grade anxiety and depression, quiet desperation, and an insidious loss of control.... It's enough to make you crazy, but seldom enough for people on the outside to validate the struggle or offer you help and respite. It's the dangerous kind of suffering—the kind that allows you to pretend that everything is OK.

This is part of the reason I kept so much of my life dissatisfaction to myself. I didn't want to sound whiny and ungrateful. A "midlife crisis" seems so damn self-indulgent, right? Hence, I often suffered alone, despite the fact that so many of us—not just a privileged few—experience what I did. Silence no more! What we're going through is normal.

I often wonder about my five friends who didn't realize that early midlife, like adolescence, is just a bridge over troubled waters. But you don't have to die and come back to life, as I did, to realize that this bridge leads to a safe shore.

Yes, your midlife unraveling can be tricky, and it requires a healthy dose of support and love from those around you. But it also offers you the first glimpses of a life less ordinary.

Seeking Your Midlife Atrium

We're living longer than ever before. Some people think this means we're going to be old longer. Anthropologist and author Mary Catherine Bateson says we're thinking about this all wrong. Our extra longevity means we're not old longer but in midlife longer. Middle age has expanded, just like our waistline. She suggests that we're not adding a metaphorical extension to our home in the form of a couple extra bedrooms in the backyard of life. We need to introduce what she calls a "midlife atrium" to support our longer lives.

Creating a midlife atrium means changing the blueprint for the whole home, or the rest of our life. This suggests we're moving the walls and, in the center of our life, creating an atrium filled with fresh air and sunlight. In a world in which some estimate that half of all children born into the developed world today will live till one hundred, it's time to re-architect our societal life blueprint by creating space for people to reflect on how to consciously curate the second half of adult life.

More than a century ago, psychologist Carl Jung asked, "Are there perhaps colleges for forty-year-olds which prepare them for their coming life and its demands as the ordinary colleges introduce our young people to a knowledge of the world?" In other words, where might we find that light-filled atrium? And are we in need of a midwife for midlife epiphanies that might emerge from this atrium?

In some ways, the sheer volume of middle-aged employees who took a break from working full-time during the COVID pandemic suggests that a collective midlife atrium is dawning. Millions of midlifers left their jobs and the cubicles that confined them and "went atrium"!

And more and more people are seeking this kind of reflection space in the company of others. Peer-to-peer midlife professional networks like Chief (for women) and Vistage are seeing huge increases in their membership. Midlife transition programs affiliated with universities, such as Stanford (Distinguished Careers Institute), Harvard (Advanced Leadership Initiative), and Notre Dame (Inspired Leadership Initiative) have grown steadily under the loose network of the Nexel Collaborative.

A version of SoulCycle, F3, pushes midlife men physically but also allows them to bond emotionally and spiritually. And even intentional communities—a communal vestige of the hippy-dippy '60s and '70s—are making a mainstream comeback focused on midlifers who are more interested in the belonging that comes from "we-tirement" than the isolation that often comes from retirement. Midlife atriums abound!

Over the past few years, I've had the great fortune of closely working with thousands of midlifers ranging in age from 28 to 88 (the average age being 54) who came to the Modern Elder Academy (MEA) to reimagine and repurpose themselves: to create a life that's as deep and meaningful as it is long.

MEA has three physical campuses—one beachfront in Baja California Sur (Mexico), one a gigantic, four-square-mile New Mexico regenerative community and horse ranch, and the last one (opening in 2026) a historic Santa Fe former Catholic seminary and retreat center. And our online campus offers deep, experiential immersions on purpose, transitions, and other topics relevant to midlifers.

MEA is the world's first midlife wisdom school that is dedicated to bringing light and space into the midlife atrium through "long-life learning." We've learned that wisdom is not taught—it's shared.

To immerse ourselves in a new community of supportive middle-aged folks who are consciously curating the second half of their lives provides an opportunity for reflection, playfulness, and growth. It's an adult summer camp, full of whimsy and wisdom. This kind of learning community—a form of encore, experiential education—will likely become more and more prevalent as people fend off the dreaded idea of retirement and reinvent themselves for the best years that lie ahead.

"There Must Be More to Life Than This"

Are you worried that you have no options, as though you've missed the last exit and have no choice but to continue pressing the pedal to the metal in a car that's running out of gas?

Life is not a one-tank journey in which you fuel up with education and relationships and a career early in life, expecting that what you've learned and experienced will provide enough energy and inspiration to last a lifetime. Life is at least a two-tank journey. To avoid getting stuck on the side of the road, we simply need to make a pit stop to refill the tank. Hopefully, this story from "down under" will inspire you.

Ang Galloway is a 53-year-old Australian who found herself at a midlife pit stop. During the first half of her life, she followed a well-worn path. School followed by university, career, marriage, kids, and divorce. It was a path that unfolded more by default than design, one that she navigated using the maps society had drawn for her rather than piloting her own direction.

During those years, Ang came to correlate servitude with success. The problem was that, after decades spent prioritizing others, she eventually forgot how to please and prioritize herself. She'd carved herself up into a thousand tiny pieces, offering a little bit to everyone, until there was nothing left.

Then the family that she had given her life to no longer required her services. One by one, they peeled off, until Ang found herself alone, inside a life she didn't recognize. A life that looked more like an empty chalk outline of what it once had been. Haunted by the ghost of the person she always dreamed she would be, she couldn't seem to shake a persistent voice that whispered, "There must be more to life than this."

Ang had filed away her youthful ambition, but within easy reach, ready to take up where she'd left off, when the time was right. Until the day she woke up and realized that the "right time" hadn't come—or if it had, she'd missed it.

By this time she had officially vacated her old life but not yet moved into her new one. A part of her was still pining for the familiarity and security that had warmed her world for the past twenty years, and a part of her felt liberated and excited by the infinite possibilities of all the unknowns that lay ahead. Ang felt simultaneously grateful for the life she had and consumed by a yearning for more. But more of what?

She knew that the blueprint for midlife and beyond that she'd inherited did not mirror the one that she wanted for herself. And yet she could not articulate what exactly she was looking for. All she knew was that she longed to rediscover the wild heart and adventurous spirit that had been dampened by societal expectations over the course of many years.

Ang says,

As a society, it's like we've won the longevity lotto, but we just haven't figured out what to do with the winnings of a longer life. It became clear that the societal roadmap I'd been referencing in my life ran out around midlife. I was betwixt and between, at a crossroads that felt both exciting and full of possibility but also terrifying and full of the unknown.

Ang said she no longer was who she was but hadn't yet become who she might be. Chrysalis, but not yet a butterfly.

She decided to design her own atrium. "What came to pass ended up being less of a plan and more of a process," she recalls. "A process of reimagining and reawakening that fueled the realization that the more abundant life I yearned for was lying dormant inside me all along, just waiting to be rediscovered and set free."

Time can be a dictator, but it can also be a liberator. Ang made the space to acknowledge and celebrate her transition from adulthood to elderhood in the form of a Golden Gap Year. It was, she says, "an opportunity to step into the unknown, full of curiosity and wonder, and reimagine what life could look like." Thus began her pilgrimage from Sydney to a rural beach town in Mexico to join a weeklong MEA workshop with a cohort of like-minded midlifers.

While midlife might feel like a solitary journey, it is often within a safe, social container that we can make space for new ways of being and knowing.

How can you find a safe crucible for life-changing conversations? A quotation often attributed to Albert Schweitzer says, "In everyone's life, at some time, our inner fire goes out. It is then burst into flame by an encounter with another human being. We should all be thankful for those people who rekindle the inner spirit." You don't have to do this alone.

How Am I Getting Happier as I Get Older?

Our societal and personal narratives of aging are at odds.

The societal message is that midlife represents the start of a long, slow death march full of disease, decrepitude, and desolation. But the U-curve of happiness research (which we'll review more in chapter 4) suggests that after a dip in life satisfaction from early adulthood that hits its bottom around 45 to 50, life gets better and happier in our 50s, 60s, 70s, and for many, even into our 80s and 90s.

Maybe the secret to happiness materializes almost automatically? Folks, just have a few more birthdays! That's not all that difficult, right?

In my daily blog, Wisdom Well, I list my Daring Dozen reasons why I'm getting happier as I get older. This list served as a kindling for the next twelve chapters of this book, in which I describe the physical, emotional, mental, vocational, and spiritual transformations that we experience in midlife. I hope this book will serve as a beacon to help you see the middle passage as the most transformative era of your life. Use it as your guide for learning to not only love midlife, but also to love *yourself* in midlife.

You may find that some chapters resonate with you more than others—whether it's no longer being defined by your body (chapter 2), appreciating your relationships more deeply (chapter 4), learning how to edit your life more rigorously (chapter 8), or stepping off the career treadmill (chapter 9). It's not essential to read them in order. Your journey through this book—as through life—is yours to define. But do spend an extra few minutes contemplating the questions in italics throughout the chapters. Think of those questions as your opportunity to experience a private personal growth workshop.

What would be on your Daring Dozen list of what gets better with age?

How are you happier and freer today than you were ten or twenty years ago?

As you've gotten older, you've learned to love brussels sprouts and classical music, so maybe it's time to learn to love midlife as well.

THE PHYSICAL LIFE

1.

"I Have More Life Left Than I Thought"

What percentage of your adult life is still ahead of you?

In 2018, I went scuba diving in Indonesia with my then 80-year-old dad. Dad learned to dive at 60 and joyfully submerged more than 2,000 times over the next 20 years, many of them in the Aquarium of the Pacific in Long Beach, California, where he regularly swam with sharks while onlookers gawked.

One morning before our first dive, I took an online longevity quiz, the results of which said I'd likely live to be 98. Wow, who knew!? Just as we were about to submerge, without letting him know I'd taken the quiz, I asked my dad how long he thought he'd live. He mused for a moment, and then to my great surprise, said, "98"!

What's miraculous about that prediction is that, if true,

my dad was barely three-quarters of the way through his adult life. And at age 57, I was not even halfway through my adult years if I lived to 98. This realization opened up doors and possibilities that have reenergized my life. Since that time, I've tried my hand (and mostly my clumsy feet) at surfing, am speaking Spanish for the first time, and have taken up pickleball (OK, I know, every person in their 60s is expected to be a pickleballer, but still). I'm convinced that when you start to realize how much life you still have ahead of you, you're more willing to try something new.

Rocky Blumhagen is a very young-looking septuagenarian friend who has always felt quite embodied. He passionately believes he's still in midlife because he'll live till 100. Rocky is super focused on preserving his body and mind. During the pandemic, he led a group of friends on Zoom through 1,000 days in a row of kundalini yoga. But Rocky had never surfed; upon coming to visit me in Mexico, he saw it as a rite of passage. It's much like learning to walk as a baby. You get up, you fall down. You get up, you fall down.

Rocky found the experience to be life-affirming, especially in his early 70s. He could apply many of his yoga principles to the experience of attuning with a wave. And the fact there was a young surfing instructor behind him reminded him that we could all use a guiding light behind us when we're trying something new and challenging, especially as we get older. He said, "The fact we were doing this as a group—all ages, colors, and sizes—gave me the added comfort and strength to get back up on my board after I'd fallen. Why don't we feel this kind of solidarity in trying something new as we age?"

Be patient when a friend in their late 40s laments about their midlife disappointment with, "How did I end up like this?" Then remind them that at that age, they're far from the "end." They haven't even hit halftime yet.

As author Jett Psaris says, "At midlife, your story is only half told." I've felt an existential impatience my whole adult life, so knowing that I may live to see my 98th birthday has helped me be more thoughtful and patient about how I design the second half of my life. At times, I feel like a young kid exploring an overflowing garden.

What's something you know or have done now that you wish you'd known or done ten years ago? Ten years from now, what will you regret if you don't learn or do it now? What's stopping you?

Anticipating your future regret—and taking steps to prevent it—is a form of wisdom that you can embrace any time in your life.

From a Three-Act to a Four-Act Play

Did you know that the characters in the *Sex in the City* sequel *And Just Like That* are the same age as the Golden Girls were when their TV series launched in 1985? Three of the Golden Girls were around 50. WTF?! On the screen, Carrie Bradshaw and her gals seem a heck of a lot younger than Betty White and Bea Arthur did! Times, fashions, and sassiness have changed, haven't they?

Twentieth-century social scientists used to look at life as though it were a three-act play, or three sets of 8,000 days, the first ending around your 21st birthday, the second ending in your mid-40s, and the last act ending around your 65th birthday, when you were retiring—and likely dying soon after that.

But, today, if you make it to 65 in the United States, there's at least a 50 percent chance you'll make it past 85; that's a whole other act, or 8,000 more days. Today, it's almost two decades later.

A century ago, you might have been dead by this age. But, today, if we live a healthy life at 50, we may get another 50 years. When we think about it this way, we realize that the core of midlife isn't the beginning of the end, but rather the long intermission of a four-act play.

Why is it that we vastly underestimate how much life we still have ahead of us? Part of it is due to our misreading of the longevity data. If we hear that American men have an average life span of 76 years old, we think that means we're going to die in less than a dozen years if we're 65 today. Yet a man who's reached 65 has added nearly 6 years to his life expectancy compared to when he was a newborn—so chances are he'll live to 82, mainly because he's survived many of the life risks of youth and early adulthood.

The older you are, the more likely you are to bust through

the longevity averages. It's time we improved our "longevity literacy."

According to a 2023 report from the TIAA Institute and George Washington University, 53 percent of midlifers surveyed are "working with inaccurate information" when it comes to life expectancy. When we underestimate our life expectancy, we are often less optimistic about the future, and less open to trying new things. When we underestimate our expiration date by a decade, we don't save enough money to afford our post-midlife years. We're not surfing or saving!

But just as we can't generalize about when midlife begins and ends, we can't generalize about longevity either, especially in the wake of the pandemic, when life spans declined in much of the world. Many variables influence how long we live, from genetics to socioeconomics to what city or part of the country we live in. In many ways, our longevity reflects not just the literal health of the country, but also its scientific advances, policy errors, and social inequities.

In midlife, we need to start distinguishing between life span and health span. The former is how long we live. The latter is *how well* we live: how long we are free from serious diseases and able to live independently. Luckily, health spans are increasing as well; in fact, if you live to be 85, you're more likely to have been active during those last 8,000 days. You don't have to age biologically as quickly as you do chronologically.

We've gotten the *quantity* part of the longevity equation generally right globally, having added thirty years to the average life span during the twentieth century. It's now time to get the *quality* part right so that people can live a life as deep and meaningful as it is long.

MEA faculty member Dan Buettner is the author of the well-known Blue Zones research that focuses on which regions of the world produce the most longevity. He cites nine variables that are most correlated with living long, healthy lives, paraphrased here:

1. Move Naturally
   The world's longest-living people garden and go for walks. They don't necessarily pump iron.
2. Have a Purpose
   Being clear about one's sense of purpose can add seven to eight years to one's life expectancy.
3. Downshift
   People with a long life span—and a long health span—incorporate practices into their daily lives that reduce stress and promote mental health.
4. Eat by the 80 Percent Rule
   Healthy agers stop eating when their stomachs are 80 percent full.
5. Eat Plants
   A plant-based diet with a limited amount of meat can extend your life several years.
6. Drink Alcohol Moderately
   People in Blue Zones drink regularly and moderately, generally with friends and/or food.

7. Belong to a Faith Community

   Attending faith-based services weekly can add four to fourteen years of life expectancy.

8. Prioritize Loved Ones

   Whether it's with blood- or chosen-family, those who live to be centenarians have deep bonds with their kin.

9. Find a Healthy Tribe

   The people who live the longest thrive in social circles that support healthy behaviors and a sense of connection.

If you're currently living in a "blah zone," living like people in a "blue zone" can extend your time on the planet. Just remember that by the time you're in midlife, the same habits that once created little noticeable damage will likely start taking a toll. Midlife is the time for us to remind ourselves that we have the power to influence how much longer we'll live.

Longevity Can Be More about Quality Than Quantity

Stanford Center on Longevity's Laura Carstensen's studies have shown that people get happier when they know they have a shorter future, as they appreciate each day more. Carstensen has also made the novel argument that we might consider abolishing retirement and instead spread periods of work, education, and sabbatical throughout our lives, thereby abandoning the tyranny of the three-stage life (learn till your early 20s, work till your early 60s, retire till you die).

Laura recently asked me if I'd be willing to give up the chance to retire in the future in exchange for a four-day workweek now. That's a provocative question and one so perfectly suited for a midlifer imagining how to curate a longer life. It's also worth considering, given the recent trend toward more flexible work.

It's surprising how many MEA alums are Millennials, given that this is a program with *Elder* in the title. Some of them are elders in their industries (e.g., a 38-year-old engineer in Silicon Valley); others are simply reconceiving the concept of midlife not as a time of crisis, but as a time of calling. Many have disavowed the three-stage life and have become experts in thinking of their lives as a series of every-ten-year sabbaticals stitched together with work in between. Others see no need for a midlife crisis because they never submitted to norms, but they also feel rocked by a less stable world.

These Millennials didn't learn the linear Game of Life board game that I did when I was a kid, back when it seemed as if there was just one path to American success. They're constantly reassessing and iterating; they march to the beat of their own drummer. Many are marrying later, having kids later, rethinking monogamy, and integrating work and life in ways we Boomers never imagined. They are the carpe diem generation. Today, many Millennials are just entering midlife—and they're doing it differently.

In some ways, I wish I could be a Millennial when I grow up. There is much I can learn from them about how to appreciate and optimize my longer life.

Are You "Age-Fluid"?

In 1981, Harvard psychologist Ellen Langer created a living time capsule. She placed study participants, most in their 70s and 80s, in an environment designed to look and feel exactly as it might have during an earlier time in their lives, when they were at the peak of their careers. Everything from the conversations to the clothing to the art, food, and music came from that era. For one week, they lived the part as if it were reality. Langer called this the "counterclockwise" experiment, because she wanted to see if giving people a chance to fully inhabit their younger selves would also turn the clock back on how old they *felt*.

It did. By the end of the one-week period, most of the participants showed marked physical and cognitive improvement. Most awakened to the fact that they actually could use skills they'd thought were lost. They showed dramatic improvements in hearing, memory, dexterity, appetite, and general well-being. It was a powerful demonstration of the saying "Age is an issue of mind over matter. If you don't mind, it doesn't matter."

I was giving a speech the other day and somehow summoned the term *age-fluid* to describe a world in which our age truly is all in our heads—a world in which fear of aging does not define us. A world in which we turn the clock back to all the ages we've ever been. In our age of gender fluidity, is age fluidity really such a stretch?

The term seemed to resonate with the audience, so after leaving the stage, I did a quick Google search. *Age-fluid* was nowhere to be found in a dictionary, except in the hipster Urban Dictionary, which had this definition: "something that justifies pedophilia."

Wow, that was so NOT what I meant! So I shelved this term for a time. But, later, when I was leading a workshop, *age-fluid* popped back up as if in a whack-a-mole game at a carnival, and people gravitated to the term again. So, in that spirit, I've decided to give it a makeover. Here goes:

Definition: "Age-fluid" (adjective): Denoting or relating to a person who does not identify themselves as having a fixed age or being part of a specific generation. Someone age-fluid might have been called "ageless" in the past. However, that definition ("never looking old or appearing to grow old") doesn't fit this context. Today's age-fluid individual is perfectly content to be both younger *and* older than their chronological age. They look at ages (or stages of life) as identities or costumes that they can don or shed.

For you age-fluid doubters, just know there are a slew of start-ups who are creating credit scores for your body. By tracking your blood, urine, and cheek swabs, they can reveal your biological age, which may be older or younger than your chronological age. And then they offer an action plan of personalized lifestyle recommendations. So, don't be surprised when you do a job interview with a candidate who convincingly tells you his driver's license says he's 60, but his doctor shows that he's 45.

In an era when you're likely to live much longer than your grandparents and you may be welcoming a less linear life, how might you become more "age-fluid"? What if you were to rethink the milestones of your life and your expectations about when they were supposed to happen? What if you gave yourself the license to live life at your own speed?

Getting Your Masters in TQ: Transitional IQ

"Human beings are works in progress that mistakenly think they're finished." So says Harvard's Dan Gilbert—and I agree. People—at all ages—vastly underestimate how much change they'll go through in their coming years. This becomes even more pronounced as we're living longer. I'm not sure Rocky would have told you 50 years ago that he'd be learning to surf in his 70s.

I don't know about you, but no one ever taught me how to master change in my life. Given our lack of education, it's no wonder we're all so apprehensive about life's transitions. Midlife is a time full of robust transitions, some of them physical, many of them psychological or spiritual. And of course, the longer we're going to live, the more opportunities for transitions we're going to have. Navigating transitions adeptly is a form of intelligence, and in midlife, building our transitional IQ (which my colleagues Jeff Hamaoui and Kari Cardinale call TQ) is essential.

When we resist a transition, we are actually resisting one or more of its three phases. We may resist *letting go* of the old; we may resist the confusion of the in-between *liminal* state (also known as the "messy middle"); or we may resist the uncertainties of a risky new *beginning*.

Chris Shore had a very stable life in suburban Indianapolis. He wasn't necessarily seeking a change from his comfortable existence. He'd married his high school sweetheart, with whom he had four children and four grandchildren by the age of 60. He had been a pastor for three dozen years and, while he enjoyed his work, he was curious about learning how to be a mentor to younger leaders, which is why he came to MEA. He did not expect his experience to set his life on a whole new course, but he came away from this experience with two new mindsets: "I do not need to be a pastor in a church to fulfill my calling, purpose, or destiny" and "I will take action to transition to my next vocation."

He returned to Indiana mulling these epiphanies, but he quickly settled back into his life and—as is true for so many of us—he wasn't sure he wanted to upset the applecart of his career at that particular moment. Then, in 2021, he was forced to confront a torrent of transitions he had neither chosen, nor prepared for: a chronic disease diagnosis (Parkinson's), an unexpected career change, and the loss of his best friend to cancer. These unforeseen events made this one of the most challenging years of his life. His faith was tested, his perspectives were challenged, and his feelings about the future were deeply conflicted.

Ironically, he had guided hundreds of others through similar storms. As a longtime pastor, he was very experienced at listening, comforting, supporting, and offering counsel to others facing health issues, unexpected life circumstances, and loss. However, he personally had been blessed with excellent health, had never been asked to leave a job, and hadn't experienced the loss of someone intimately close to him since his grandparents died, years before.

Chris was blindsided by a new church leader's decision to eliminate his position and move the church in a new direction. He was in the precarious place of being 60 and jobless, with a résumé that included only pastoral ministry in a church. Fortunately, some members of his congregation saw his value as a seasoned leader, and he is now working for a growing company in the corporate world. This was not an easy transition, but one that brought him new energy and joy and proved that he could evolve.

Throughout the dense fog of change, it was Chris's TQ that helped him see the path to his new life and bid adieu to a past that had sustained him but was no longer nourishing him. While he's still wary about his health condition, he plans to live a few more decades, so his awareness of the three stages of any transition will serve him the rest of his life.

Life is inherently liminal, often leaving us feeling as if

we have no firm footing. It's awkward to feel unmoored in midlife, but it's normal. Midlife is a time full of surprises and challenges. Yet learning to embrace the liminal opens one up to so many new choices.

Here are three questions to consider if you want to increase your TQ as you increase your life expectancy:

1. *What can you learn from your childhood self?* As a child you navigated learning to walk, going through puberty, romance—perhaps getting dumped by your first love, feeling out of place in a new job. Yes, you were awkward during these times, but you got through them. What can you learn from how you coped? Are you better able to navigate your liminal periods today than when you were younger and, either way, why?

2. *Are you in the caterpillar, the chrysalis, or the butterfly stage of your transitions?* Understanding which stage you're in will give you the self-awareness to be patient with yourself. For the caterpillar, ritualizing is essential to ending something. Time in the chrysalis helps you find the narrative thread between old and new and make sense of the messy middle. Embracing the fun in being a beginner is the best strategy for emerging as a butterfly to enter your new beginning.

3. *Is perfectionism or impatience getting in your way?* Author Bruce Feiler's work shows that the average adult transition takes three to five years, so don't expect to emerge from the chrysalis overnight. There are tricks to

accelerating the metamorphosis process, but being perfect isn't one of them.

"Don't Give Up at Halftime"

Legendary Alabama football coach Bear Bryant famously said, "Don't give up at halftime." Good advice for us all. How are you preparing for the second half of your adult life? If the first half was learning the rules, could the second half be about breaking them? And one of the key rules to break is the societal mindset that midlife is boring and uninspired. Break convention. Break habits. Break free!

You're likely to live a helluva long time. How might you design your life differently knowing how much life you have ahead of you?

Are you willing to take a gap year, at minimum, once per decade until the end of your working life?

If you could go back to school for a year, what subject would you study and how might you utilize that knowledge in your life?

How would you live if you knew you had only five to ten years left?

How would you live if you knew you were going to live until 100?

2.

"I'm Relieved My Body No Longer Defines Me"

Just as I got comfortable in my own skin,
it started to sag.

Our obsession with getting older is so focused on the physical, on how it looks, that we don't prepare for what it *feels* like to experience midlife.

Aging is a privilege, a gift of time. Yet so many of us focus our middle-age conversations on what we have lost: we share "organ recitals" of what body parts no longer work as they used to and long for our youthful beauty and brawn. If we made space to age in a more natural way, free of the external pressures regarding how we look, how much more pleasurable could midlife be?

Let's acknowledge that aging is something we do in public. We can hide other facts about ourselves, but we wear our age with shame, with pride, or with touch-ups. No matter how artfully a face has been adorned or a hairline has been restored, it is obvious to all that an older person inhabits this image. How we feel about our longevity is on display, not only in our attempts at concealment but in how we embrace or resist our additional years. And, of course, midlife is when our body makes its presence known in all kinds of aches, pains, and health conditions.

If this sounds just awful, then you're likely still living your life on the playing field of the body. You may judge your self-worth based upon how you used to look or what you think 50 should look like (which is a lot different than it used to be). There are so many other playing fields you could be enjoying: the playing field of your heart, your soul, your mind, your community.

It's ironic that in midlife we become more comfortable in our own skin just as it starts to sag. This can freak people out. So, just as we've diligently filled our calendar in our 30s and 40s, some of us start to do the same in filling every crease on our face. We don't seem to appreciate that we've earned those wrinkles. Let me tell you the story of someone who decided she wasn't going to play on that playing field of the body anymore.

The Half-Trillion-Dollar Anti-Aging Industry

Tara Gadomski is an actor, filmmaker, and radio producer. You may have seen her on *Orange Is the New Black* or on *The*

Blacklist. As someone who's worked in Hollywood, she's acutely aware of how women have the odds stacked against them as they age.

Tara found that sometime in her mid-40s, she stopped being terrified of wrinkles. Until then, she had followed all the expert advice on how to fight them. Some rules were basic—like always using SPF. Others required a bit more invest-ment—like sleeping on a silk pillowcase. Then there were the rules that were downright strange—like placing tape between her eyebrows while at home, to stop her face from forming any expression that might develop into a crease over time.

She says,

> There isn't a particular "aha" moment that stopped me from being afraid, but rather, it was a gradual awakening to the idea that we are being told a false narrative—that young, thin, able-bodied, and white is the ideal look. And this false narrative exists to make us buy things. Once I stopped being afraid, I got mad. I was angry that the $571-billion-dollar global "beauty" industry had led me to believe, my whole life, that I was "flawed" and needed to be "corrected," with a product.

Welcome to the anti-aging industrial complex obsessed with keeping us youthful, when what really matters is remain-ing useful. And, of course, this industry might as well be called anti-women because that's the target market, with the bull's-eye on their back. It's alarming how the age at which women (and men) are getting Botox and plastic surgery is growing younger and younger. It's almost as if the ultimate compliment is "You don't look a day over 30," so people try to capture that age and hold on to it with an iron grip...or iron face, no less.

Let's also recognize the fact that there's a vanishingly narrow band of time when a woman is viewed as neither too young and inexperienced, nor too old, washed up, or "past her prime." As a friend of mine noted, "At 35, people dismissed me in my career for being too young and, yet, by 40, I no longer thought it was wise to have kids. Somehow, the totality of my adult life was supposed to be wedged into the 5 years in between. It was a time when I was stressed and exhausted."

For women approaching the early stage of midlife, anxiety around aging may be tied to the biological clock ticking inside them. Research has shown they're likely to feel on schedule or off schedule. Men, however, don't have the pressure of this timeline. In fact, society seems to appreciate the soul-searching man who's taking his time to find himself before settling down and starting a family. But most women simply aren't afforded the luxury of doing such things on their own time.

The male midlife crisis is the stuff of clichés and late-night jokes (don't worry, men, we'll get to you in a moment). The female version, however, is talked about much less. There's an invisibility that many women feel as they age. It's not just that the dating odds are typically skewed against middle-aged women; it's also that men simply don't notice them in the same way. And however unwelcome the attention might have been in their 20s and 30s, its absence is felt in a palpable way. And while Hollywood has labeled George Clooney and Richard Gere "silver foxes," we don't have the same affection for aging leading ladies. "Silver vixen" is not a similarly common term, and very few women appreciate being characterized as a "cougar."

Thank God for Emma Thompson, who in the 2022 film *Good Luck to You, Leo Grande*, offers a coming-of-age tale of a straight-arrow woman in her early 60s, who falls for a handsome, young biracial male prostitute and realizes that it's time to give sex another chance. In the very last scene of the film, she stares at herself in the mirror, stark naked. Having admired her emotional nakedness throughout the film, seeing Thompson's "full monty" is no shock to the viewer. What's powerful is how you can feel her revelation that she's no longer defined by her body.

Men are not spared the bodily indignities of aging. Because the male version of menopause—known as andropause—is less well-known (and less disruptive), men tend to deny all their physical foibles when they're often quite natural. A loss of virility. A growing gut. Getting winded doing the same exercise you did so easily ten years ago. While women tend to share their feelings about the physical by-products of time, men hold them inside.

Too many of us are living with an outdated paradigm about aging, based upon our relationship with our bodies. According to this narrative, we peak in early midlife, and then it's one long, slow rot. But in midlife, we realize that the playing field of life has moved from the body to the heart and soul. Aristotle recognized this progression long ago; he believed the body was perfect at 35 and the soul at 49.

Initially, this was a tough pill to swallow for my MEA cofounder Christine Sperber, a self-described "ski bum turned cofounder." That's what she wrote in her bio for a business conference she was attending, but truth be told, Christine was once a professional snowboarder who rode the half pipe for money. She earned her living with her body, with her physical skill and strength. Now she's long retired, but she still hangs out on the slopes. Christine knows that to avoid injury, she has to invest in Pilates, stretching, and stamina training more than in the past.

She is no stranger to physical pain, however. As a young FIS World Cup competitor, she was constantly sore from pushing herself past her limits every single day. It was good, worthy pain. She was paid to travel the world and to regularly loosen gravity's grip on her body by propelling herself up a snow wall and careening into the air beyond the edge of the half pipe, at amazing speeds.

But, at 53 years old, Christine has found the physical toll of perimenopause to be nearly as daunting as boarding on the slopes. It's affected her sleep, her skin, her hair and she's had a steady spree of hot flashes and migraines. And she's curious about why no one talks about this natural transition that women experience. She laments, "The fact that every woman I've known in my entire life traveled this way and not a word nor a whisper about this was shared, that migraines are a common symptom and my doctor never mentioned that as a possibility—it's all shocking to me."

She's always been her body. But she has had to come to terms with the fact that what was once her livelihood is, at midlife, just a hobby. She says the joy and the freedom of snowboarding are inexplicable to the uninitiated, and she'll continue to do it until she can't. The transition from athlete to middle-aged business person wasn't easy, but it is one she is grateful for. She continues, "The young athlete 'me' might be shocked that I would be paid for my ideas—that my body, while softening, would simply be the carrier for my brain, ever sharpening." Cultural anthropologist Margaret Mead suggested that this era of life could be full of "postmenopausal zest."

Too often, we think of aging as a slow decline of the human body. But perhaps a more appropriate metaphor, as Jane Fonda has suggested, is "a staircase, symbolizing the upward ascension of the human spirit, bringing us into wisdom, wholeness, and authenticity."

I would suggest it's a spiral staircase, which allows us a 360-degree opportunity—unobstructed by blind spots of our youth—to become "first-class noticers" of all that's below. Through willpower, courage, resilience, humor, self-awareness, the support of others guiding you, and possibly faith, we gain access to the stunning view that comes with our later years. We earn that view with hard work, wisdom, and our willingness to keep climbing.

What Does a Six-Pack Cost You?

The older you are, the more expensive a six-pack.

No, I'm not talking about the $10 to $12 you shell out for six Budweisers. I'm referring to the six-pack abs that our culture reveres. Here's a statistic for all you guys loafing on the couch. For affluent women (making more than $150,000 per year), a man's abs are the number one body feature they focus on. And, when asking all women, no matter their earnings, abs are more important than the eyes, face, legs, and many other body parts. As well, the thousands of ads depicting shirtless men and the disparaging jokes about "dad bods" also have middle-aged men preoccupied with their six-packs. It's no wonder men get a little fixated on their tummies as they age.

I have a friend (to remain unnamed) who added his "COVID-19" weight almost exclusively to his gut and was obsessed about it. He was on a mission to get back to the six-pack he had in his 20s, and he knew that he had to lose 10 to 20 percent of his body fat to get there. I took the liberty of doing the math for him. If he loses 1 to 2 percent of body fat per month on a combo diet and serious workout regime, it'll probably take him a year to get his six-pack back. Twenty years ago, it would have taken him half as long. And we're not even talking about the effort it would take to keep off the weight.

But here's where the real cost of that six-pack comes in. The dude is no fun anymore! (Don't worry, he knows it.) He's obsessed with his scorecard on physical aging. He no longer grabs a drink with friends after work. My Zoom calls with him happen while he's walking on his home treadmill. And he spends so much time thinking about diet and exercise, he's lost interest in a variety of topics we used to discuss: politics, racial injustice, travel, and where to get pizza!

Philosopher Henry David Thoreau says that "the cost of a thing is the amount of...life which is required to be exchanged for it, immediately or in the long run." Based upon this definition of cost, I'd say my friend's six-pack is crazy expensive.

To be fair, men have a challenge regarding belly fat that women don't have. About 90 percent of our body fat is "subcutaneous fat" that is more of an evenly distributed layer. The rest is "visceral fat," which is found deeper in the body, behind abdominal muscles. It collects in the abdominal cavity and poses more serious health risks than subcutaneous fat, as it can affect our organs. Men are more likely to accumulate visceral fat, especially when our hormones start to change during andropause. So, men, it's worth giving this attention—without being obsessive about it.

Now don't get me wrong. I'm all for staying healthy and looking good. But, as we age, we also have to remember that time is our most precious resource and then ask *Is the cost worth it?*

Well-known executive coach and author Alisa Cohn believes it is. But her investment in her body isn't a vanity project; it's about health. Growing up in a small Massachusetts town, she was a self-described "sit-on-the-couch-and-read kind of girl." Her mom was heavy, her family was not active, and she grew up in a community that got together over large meals, not bike rides or hikes. When she was 17, she decided she had to make a change. She put on her little Tretorn sneakers and ran up the street. Three minutes later, she was lying on the floor of her living room, hyperventilating. So she had... let's call it an *uneasy relationship* with fitness.

As a young adult, Alisa began to understand that she had the power to intentionally shape her own life. She was also lucky to have a bossy therapist, who told her that she had to either commit to rigorous physical activity or see a psychiatrist about antidepressants. She chose the former. She started going to the gym three days a week, where she learned that physical activity would reliably turn a bad mood around.

"I began to be pulled towards fitness by a carrot," she remembers. "I joined a running group and a cycling group. I loved being part of those communities, being outside, being fit. I ended up running three half-marathons, and after each one I gave an emotional high-five to that teenager lying on the floor, out of breath. It was a triumph over my past."

Alisa is right. Healthy aging requires us to move our bodies. Fitness is about more than just our physical health; it's about the ability to do fun things for our entire lives — traveling, taking a stroll through the park, chasing little kids around the yard — as well as essential things like carrying heavy groceries into the house, shoveling the driveway, and walking up three flights of stairs if the elevator is broken.

Here's maybe the most important question of this chapter. Answer it honestly, please. What's prompting your investment in your body? Is it investing in your long-term health or in your short-term vanity?

Middlescence: The Adult Corollary to Adolescence

Let me introduce you to a word that you've probably never heard of, but one that's very relevant to what is going on with your body in midlife.

Respected gerontologists, Ken Dychtwald and Barbara Waxman, have been popularizing the word *middlescence* to describe the life stage that has emerged out of increased longevity patterns in the twenty-first century.

The last time a word describing a life stage entered the mainstream global lexicon was in the 1890s, when *adolescence* increasingly entered popular discussion. In 1904, psychologist G. Stanley Hall published a book titled *Adolescence*, in which he describes the teens and early 20s as a time of "storm and stress." Today, we recognize adolescence as a time when we experience major transitions, both physically (puberty) and emotionally (our sense of who we are and how we see the world). In earlier centuries, society rushed kids into adulthood at what now seems like an alarmingly early age; marriage, babies, and farmwork or a job in a factory all might happen before the end of puberty. Fortunately, we now see adolescence as a necessary and natural preparatory course for adulthood.

Maybe it's time for a similar rethinking of midlife, a time

when our bodies—and identities—are changing once again. As we did in our teens, we're going through profound physical, hormonal, emotional, and existential transitions during this time. So much of this change is focused on our bodies.

Middlescence is a time of endings and beginnings. Yet, while we have all kinds of rituals to support and recognize adolescents during their transitional time of life (bar/bat mitzvahs, communion, quinceañera, high school graduation, etc.), little is provided for middlescence. Where are the midlife ceremonies or opportunities for merrymaking to mark our passage, to make the space to reflect on and audit our life experience to repurpose it in new ways?

Middlescence can also offer a newfound experience of sexuality. For some, there is relief in the fact that there's no longer the risk of an unwanted pregnancy. For some men, it's when they feel they've been let out of testosterone prison. For others, sensuality starts to emerge as the unexpected "bedfellow." And still others find it's the time when their long-practiced skill at people-pleasing comes full circle to themselves.

Author John Updike suggests that midlife is marked by "insatiable egos and workable genitals" which can lead to rampant adultery. But perhaps that's an immature view of middlescence. More often than not, this is an era when we settle into a less performative, more relaxed rhythm with a partner.

Too many of us have the misconception that biology is the only predictor of sexual health as we age, so we turn to hormones and prescriptive medications. But the self-awareness and desire to connect on a deeper, intimate level that comes with age can create even greater sensual satisfaction than that we experienced earlier in our adulthood.

Middlescence may be the first time in your life when you fall in love with your body just the way it is.

Is My Body Failing Me, or Am I Failing My Body?

I can't say I've fallen in love with my body the past few years as the question rolling around my brain has been "Am I the victim or the perpetrator?" More than five years into my prostate cancer journey, I've come to realize that my relationship between the victim (me) and the perpetrator (the disease) is codependent.

I was in seemingly excellent health when I got the news that I had intermediate-stage prostate cancer in 2018, so it came as a surprise. My immediate response was to spend the next year trying to be a hero to my body: working with a functional medicine doctor, changing my diet, going to a weeklong cleansing and fasting spa, drinking green juice, taking supplements every morning, and exercising and meditating more. The good news is my cancer went dormant and, other than the active surveillance through regular testing, the tumultuous relationship between my body and the disease became copacetic.

Then the pandemic came along, and all bets were off. I started eating too much dark chocolate and drinking too much alcohol as coping mechanisms during a stressful time. I also became delinquent about my prostate testing because, well, my doctor was in San Francisco, and I was stuck in paradise (Baja), given travel restrictions. More than anything, I'd forgotten that food and drink are a form of medicine. Long story short, three years after my diagnosis, my cancer started growing again, which led to a surgery in which I lost half my prostate, followed by a reinvigorated health regimen.

Post-surgery, when I was told that there was only a one percent chance that the cancer would metastasize within five years, it felt like I could coast a little again...until I found out 15 months later that the cancer had spread to my lymphatic system. So now it was time for hormone therapy and taking out the rest of my prostate. It would have been easy to feel resentful or angry at my body for failing me, but today, I'm focused less on who is to blame and more on a truth and reconciliation approach to restoring my health. My body and I are in a partnership.

I've become an enlightened witness to the deterioration and regeneration of my body. Society looks at aging as linear — one long, slow decline — but the reality is that it's cyclic, as our body is constantly regenerating itself. Our skin renews itself every month. Our stomach lining every five days. Our body is rebuilding itself each and every year based upon how we treat it.

I've learned that cancer can have a silver lining. It can become a rite of passage, an invitation to a form of self-transformation. Rather than see my body as a vanity vehicle, the physical manifestation of my ego, I now see it as a trusted best friend. We're not always in sync, but I assume the best intentions of my body, and it holds me accountable when I've neglected it. It is not a machine to be optimized, but instead a friend to be loved.

What if your body isn't at war with you? What if your body is your wisest teacher, guiding you to the truths you need to learn? Before going to bed each night, maybe you can ask your wise body, "How can you teach me to live a better life?"

Creating a New Relationship with Your Body

So you've spent most of your life creating the container—your body—that defines how you see yourself and how the world sees you. It's time to realize that you are more than your body and your looks. Yes, others may notice your aging more than you do, especially when you show up at your first college reunion in a decade. So what?! Everyone else at that reunion is in a similarly creaky old boat, like you.

As we discussed earlier, given how much life you still have ahead of you, don't forget about your body, but don't obsess about it either. Think about the activities you want to be able to do when you're 90 and then recognize that if those things require physical strength and agility—and they do—you need to start to train for them now.

In sum, love your body. It's a rental vehicle you were issued at birth, and you may have forty to fifty years ahead of you.

That's a lot of mileage for your banged-up vehicle. Some of us maintain our vehicle with tender loving care and precision, while others drive like the Baja 1000 off-road motorsport race. Along the way, we all need a few pit stops, as well as a skillful road crew for whatever conditions we may face.

But, just as a car depreciates with time, so does your body. It's being reclaimed by nature as you grow older. Nature is asserting her rights to decompose you. It's not a curse. It may even be a blessing as it helps you to experience so much more than bodily pleasures and egoic mirror gazing. Beauty is more than skin deep. And as we'll see in the next couple of chapters, it's our emotions and our relationships that sustain us in our later years.

THE EMOTIONAL LIFE

3.

"I'm Making Friends with My Emotions"

*As we grow older, real beauty moves from
the face to the heart.*

I loathed two notions when I was younger: to be *content* and to be *settled*. Both of them felt like compromises. Seeking contentment and comfort sounded so damn ordinary. It reminded me of something my radical tenth-grade history teacher taught me: "Comfort breeds apathy." And feeling settled sounded like just this side of what happens in a coffin.

More recently, I've realized that happiness is the playing field of youth, and contentment (even joy) is the reward of later life. I'm reminded of an inscription that appears on a seventeenth-century stone basin in Kyoto, Japan, translated sometimes as "What I have is all I need" or "I am content with what I am."

Happiness is not the same thing as joy; as author J. D.

Salinger—who lived to 91—has written that "happiness is a solid and joy a liquid." Happiness is often based upon external circumstances, but joy bubbles up from inside you.

Midlife is when we start to realize that happiness does not consist of the gratification of our wishes. It is a choice made in the mind, not in the gym. When it comes to our "pursuit of happiness," we don't always appreciate or revel in what we already have. In the first half of our life, we often pursue gratification rather than practicing gratitude.

Research has shown that we grow more satisfied with life after age 50. And this isn't just an American thing, as researchers have found this U-curve of happiness to be nearly universal across countries. It's not because all our problems magically melt away. Instead, it's because we learn to roll with the punches and gracefully accept the unexpected assaults of life and not take them personally. Our obsession with "more, more, more" has subsided. And in its place is an ability to welcome the joy of the simplest gifts—a smile from a stranger, a new book on our bedside table, a thoughtful gesture from our friend or spouse.

Five Signs Your EQ Is Improving with Age

What if the secret to being happier was purely just to get older? Sounds absurd, right?

Society tells us that midlife is a time of regret, frustration, and sadness. But the reality is that we actually experience *less* of these things as we age. Who knew that life cycles of happiness and contentment were so natural and predictable?

Why does the happiness curve decline from early adulthood before swinging upward around age 45 to 50? The early stage of midlife can often feel less like a midlife crisis and more like a midlife circus. The spinning plates. The whining kids and dying parents. The career woes. No time for friends, fun, or frolicking (especially in the bedroom). We may begin to feel like we need a Container Store for our damn emotions.

At the same time, however, we finally have the tools to handle what life throws at us. By 50, our EQ (emotional IQ) is higher than it's ever been. We've seen enough good and bad times to understand what coping skills work for us. We've started practicing "psycho-hygiene" rituals—ways of living that cleanse our minds and hearts. We realize that we are more resilient than we ever thought. Ideally, we've learned to dance with our emotions instead of shoving them in a drawer.

UC Berkeley psychologist Robert Levenson is one of many academics who has demonstrated that while IQ stays relatively stable during one's adulthood, EQ rises with time. Levenson's team studied a group of research subjects who ranged in age from their 20s to their 60s. He asked them to watch a series of video clips designed to elicit different emotions, such as disgust and sadness, then try to modulate their emotions in response to the nasty or heart-rending clips—either to remain unmoved or to try to see the upside of whatever they witnessed on-screen.

Which age group was best able to tap into their emotional responses?

The researchers found that the older the participant, the better they were at both reinterpreting the scenes in positive ways—a technique called "positive reappraisal"—and at actively processing the emotions the video clips elicited: a hallmark sign of emotional intelligence. That's because, as he explains it, "Evolution seems to have tuned our nervous systems in ways that are optimal for these kinds of interpersonal and compassionate activities as we age."

Furthermore, Penn State University psychologist David Almeida has been studying the daily stressors of more than 3,000 adults for the past thirty years. He's shown that people in early adulthood may report stressors on at least 40 to 45 percent of days, but by the time they're in later midlife, that goes down to maybe 20 to 25 percent of days. Part of this is due to our ability to reframe and digest our normal day-to-day challenges.

OK, now let's move from the scientists to the practitioners—in other words, us. Here are my observations on how my EQ has grown with age so that I see my emotions as friends, not enemies:

1. **I feel more compassion for others.** As I age, I've softened...and not just around my belly. I experience less ego and more soul. And I feel more deeply for others' life circumstances. Fortunately, I am able to direct some of that increased compassion toward myself as well.

2. **I am less emotionally reactive and more emotionally fluent.** When I was younger, I had a kind of emotional vertigo; my emotions constantly made me feel imbalanced and uneasy. I didn't know how to dance with them. In fact, I often tried to outrun my emotions. Today, I'm more emotionally fluent and my emotions have moderated, partly because I've learned not to sweat the small stuff. Like the older participants in Levenson's study, I'm able to "positively reappraise" negative experiences, like getting stuck in traffic in an Uber (interpretation: great chance to meditate). Simultaneously, my enhanced ability to recognize my patterns, habits, and tendencies allows me to observe myself more effectively.

3. **I don't take things so personally.** Don Miguel Ruiz, the author of *The Four Agreements*, says, "There is a huge amount of freedom that comes to you when you take nothing personally." This skill is particularly valuable in our polarized, "cancel culture" era.

4. **I have a better understanding of how to create my ideal habitats.** Social scientists call this "environmental mastery," the ability to determine which environments one will flourish in—and the capacity to adjust and adapt to changes in those habitats. This also speaks to why, in the workplace, older people on a team have been found to create more "psychological safety" on teams: because their environmental mastery, combined with their compassion, helps them create the proper conditions for team flourishing.

5. **I value relationships more.** It's been said that the two questions people ask on their deathbed are "Did I love well, and was I well-loved?" The longitudinal Harvard Study on Adult Development and the Blue Zones research conclusively show that the relationships we cultivate in our lives can actually increase our life span. We'll talk more about that in the next chapter.

Of course, there are always outliers—Exhibit A: your perennially grumpy 75-year-old uncle. But he's an exception, not the rule. The research shows that if you focus on developing your emotional intelligence, you will also develop another kind of EQ—*Enhanced Quality* of life. And that's an EQ we can all appreciate, especially as we age.

Living with a Broad Margin of Error

When we're young, we tend to live our lives within a tiny margin of error. We overestimate the cost of failure (especially our own), and we retreat into a fixed mindset. In midlife, many of us finally learn to cut ourselves some slack. We no longer refuse to play the games that we aren't sure we can win. We can focus on *improving* ourselves instead of just *proving* ourselves.

Did you grow up thinking that you were defined by your successes and failures? I know I sure did. So much of my adolescent self-worth came from my achievements. Of course, it isn't healthy to attach your self-esteem to your success at any age, but doing so gets even more treacherous as we get older. If you play only games you can win, your sandbox gets smaller and smaller.

There's been substantive research showing that a growth mindset is one of the keys to successful aging. For those with a growth mindset, success isn't defined by winning but, instead, learning. A growth mindset facilitates seeking out, exploring, and enjoying new experiences. It is the antidote to midlife boredom.

A growth mindset also can be helpful in our normal daily rituals. For example, when it comes to sleep, I was stuck in a fixed mindset for decades: "I'm someone who never sleeps well." Until, in my mid-50s, I tried on a growth mindset: "I wonder what might help me sleep better." I now sleep more than an hour longer each night than I used to—thanks to some helpful natural supplements such as magnesium and melatonin and better sleep practices (going to bed around the same time on both weekdays and weekends).

"In my 40s," writes author Jonathan Rauch in his essay, "The Real Roots of Midlife Crisis," "I found I was obsessively comparing my life with other people's: scoring and judging myself and counting up the ways in which I had fallen behind in an unwinnable race: *Why don't I have as many zeros in my bank account as Jeff Bezos? Or Barack Obama is younger than me, and look where he is!*"

I can relate. One of my greatest midlife lessons has been that comparison is the recipe for suffering; that is, until a growth mindset helped me to peel off the bumper sticker in my mind that said I was bad at yoga.

I learned to meditate in my early 20s when I was going through a stressful time. I took to meditation immediately, partly because I found it easy to close my eyes and inhabit my inner world. Yoga, on the other hand, was a struggle for me for decades, primarily because for this activity, my eyes were open, staring at a room full of California yoginis who seemed to be able to place their legs behind their heads while standing up. I felt like a "stiff upper Chip": more lumber than limber.

It wasn't till a few years ago that I realized what was triggering my fixed mindset of "I'm terrible at yoga." It was social comparison: how I looked to others, not how I felt inside my own body. So, for the past few years, I've been doing one-on-one yoga instruction with our MEA mindfulness teacher, Teddi Dean, at my home. No one is watching but Teddi and my dog, Jamie, who does not trigger this particular insecurity despite her mastery of the downward dog position. Now I feel much more comfortable and less self-conscious even in a yoga class with others. Plus, I'm less focused on striving to make it "look right."

Douglas Tsoi, 50, the founder of the School of Financial Freedom, has had an unconventional career, ranging from corporate law to spiritual direction. Not long ago, he shared a revelation he had while stretching after a soccer game, leaning up against his dog and basking in the sun. He was so grateful for what life afforded him: financial security, a working body, and time to enjoy life. Time to learn and do important things, enjoy yummy foods, and love the beauty of living in the Pacific Northwest.

He says, "I realized that MY job is to be grateful for MY life, for the things I have." It was the "particular-ness" of his gratitude, he said, that shielded him from either envy or pride.

What would a "Day without Envy or Comparison" feel like? A day in which you settled into the gifts of your own life, with not a care in the world about how they compare with others. If you can muster a day of bliss, maybe you can stretch it to a week, a month, a year, or a lifetime. Here's one way to summon up some gratitude. Ask yourself, "Who made it possible to be who I am and do what I'm doing right now?"

Gratitude without self-judgment: a prescription for a contented life.

Becoming Who You're Meant to Be

Isidra Mencos is a Spanish-American woman who felt lost in early midlife. She was born and raised in Barcelona, Spain, where she spent her 20s experimenting with the new freedoms afforded by the end of the Franco dictatorship. She was, in her own words, "bouncing from man to man and job to job"; she freelanced for prestigious publishing houses, traveled the world as a tour leader, and worked for the Olympic Committee.

In 1992, she came to the U.S. to earn a PhD in Spanish and Latin American Contemporary Literature. She was accepted by several universities and chose UC Berkeley, because it sounded bohemian. After graduating, she taught, freelanced, and worked a corporate gig as an editorial director. But none of her jobs were truly satisfying, as she felt disconnected from her calling.

Isidra felt like she was always arriving late to everything important, even though she was obsessively punctual in her everyday life. She became a rebellious teenager in her early 20s—a full decade behind schedule—after a fairly tame adolescence. She didn't have what she called "a real career" until her late 30s. By the time she got married, most of her childhood friends had been hitched for over a decade; when she became a mother, their kids were already in high school. And she was still an "emerging writer" while the writer friends from her youth rested on the laurels of their literary awards. Comparison could have been her recipe for suffering.

Instead, she looked at her late blooming life as a gift, a prolonged opportunity to learn about who she was meant to be. Some of these insights arrived via dreams, conflicts, or tensions, synchronicities, and meditation, and even through some health challenges.

She shared one story with me:

I had a vision in my early twenties. I saw an old Chinese man with a long, flowing white beard and hair climb up a mountain. When he reached the top, he played his flute. The beautiful melody ascended to the clouds, flew to the peaks of the surrounding mountains, and cascaded into the valley below. I knew instantly this man was me and the music was my writing. I was meant to share my voice and my art with the world. But I resisted my calling, burying it deep into my shadow. I was scared to be rejected and unheard.

It was only in midlife that Isidra had the emotional intelligence, and the courage, to become the writer she'd always meant to be. Yes, at times, she regrets that she didn't find her true writing voice earlier, but she says she has so much more to say now that she's lived a more seasoned life. Here's a poetic thought often attributed to Anaïs Nin that reminds her that being a late bloomer is better than not blooming at all: "The day came when the risk to remain tight in the bud became more painful than the risk it took to blossom."

Knowing Your Own Mind and Heart Is Your Superpower

After a lifetime of being joined at the hip with Chip, I have become an expert in my own emotions. Emotional intelligence can be a heady topic, but at the end of the day, it just means we become a sage counselor, best friend, and partner, both to ourselves and to others.

The ultimate middle-aged skill is knowing what you want from life. We spend so much of our first half of adulthood taste-testing life based upon conventional wisdom, social pressure, and family obligation. No wonder we make so many ill-guided decisions about love, work, family, and friends up through our 40s.

Understanding what you truly want will get you further in life than talent or hard work. It gives you agency, and when you feel that kind of influence over your life, you can handle disappointment when it arises, because you realize you acted on no one's terms but your own. Once you know what you want *from* life, you are better able to give back *to* life.

So much of how we live our early adulthood has been prescribed by others. I grew up with the Ten Commandments as my guide for "living a good life," and I'm guessing many of you did, too. They always felt very negative to me. A heckuva lot of "shalt nots." In fact, eight of the ten tell us what NOT to do.

So, in midlife, I chose to create "My Ten Commitments" based upon my newfound understanding of what I'm committed TO do. These have proven to be my emotional guides of how I choose to live my life. I don't think I could have developed a list like this when I was 30:

1. I commit to living a life more focused on my eventual eulogy than my current résumé.
2. I show up with a passionate engagement in life because, that way, people will notice my energy more than my wrinkles.
3. I assume best intentions in people, unless they've been proven untrustworthy.

4. I follow the old adage "Live as if you were going to die tomorrow. Learn as if you were going to live forever."
5. I try to be curious, not judgmental (subscribing to the Ted Lasso school of philosophy).
6. I seek "noble experiments" that will help me discover something new (even though I will likely make lots of mistakes).
7. I learn from my mistakes because that's how I grow my wisdom.
8. I embrace my emotions, as they're my best evidence that I'm human.
9. I don't chase happiness. I practice gratitude, and happiness is the natural result.
10. I remember that my most valuable sense is my sense of humor, as it's something I still possess even if I've lost everything else.

Could you find some time to craft your own Ten Commitments that will guide your emotional response to life?

While our life circumstances don't necessarily get easier as we age, our responses to them drastically improve. We are less reactive, more self-aware, and our capacity for empathy soars. Who wouldn't find this era of life an improvement over our earlier decades?

4.

"I Invest in My Social Wellness"

Illness starts with the letter I, while Wellness starts with the letters We.

In the midst of the pandemic lockdowns, we saw videos of Italians singing from their apartment balconies to deserted streets and family members half-heartedly celebrating at Zoom weddings and funerals finding the virtual version of these rituals an unsatisfying substitute for the real thing. At the end of the pandemic, we saw that social distancing was swiftly replaced with social visiting, as the first trips most people took were to see friends and family that they'd missed. We're wired with an urge to merge, aren't we?

When most of us think of wellness, we often think of it as a personal effort, not something we experience together (nope, your Peloton class at home is not a form of social wellness).

What if we began to look at our wellness as a shared responsibility, striving for social, not just personal wellness.

Maybe it's time to count NOT how many steps we took or how many calories we consumed, but how many sunsets we experienced with our spouse, how many times we felt goose bumps during a deep conversation with our best friend, or how many times we smiled at a stranger?

I regularly count the magnificent waves where I live here in this small fishing and farming beachfront village of Baja California Sur, Mexico. I'm not talking about the towering waves in the ocean, but the hand waves I receive from locals when I drive down our dusty, bumpy roads. Waving hello is standard practice here — one that builds community and heals.

In midlife, we start to gain a little distance from our own importance, so that we see the panorama of moral and natural beauty all around us. It is in these moments that we often feel most alive, and it's most inspiring when it's in the company of others. If we're lucky, we feel a "collective effervescence" when our sense of individual ego evaporates and our communal joy emerges.

How Well Are You Living?

In 1938, researchers at Harvard created one of the best-known social science projects of all time: a stunningly ambitious attempt to answer the question of what makes a person thrive over the course of a lifetime. Every five years since, the researchers gathered detailed physical and emotional health records on the 724 participants. Eighty-five years later, the

Harvard Study of Adult Development is the longest-running study on human happiness in the world.

A few years ago, I was introduced to Dr. Robert Waldinger, who runs the longitudinal study. His research on how to live a good life struck a chord; his TED talk has been viewed more than 40 million times and his most recent book, with coauthor Marc S. Schulz, *The Good Life: Lessons from the World's Longest Scientific Study of Happiness*, was a bestseller. While many of us believe that being rich, famous, talented, or powerful is the superhighway to happiness, Dr. Waldinger says that the surest path to contentment is more like a country road.

What makes the Harvard Study of Adult Development so unprecedented is the fact that they have been able to study this research cohort over the course of a long lifetime. And while there were many conclusions to emerge, one thing stood out above the rest: that good relationships keep us happier and healthier — particularly as we age.

"Repeatedly, when the participants in our study reached old age," the authors write in *The Good Life*, "they would make a point to say that what they treasured most were their relationships." While younger adults benefit from having a large number of less intimate friendships, the study showed, as we get older, it's the quality, not the quantity, of the relationships that matters.

So how is this relevant to you in midlife? The researchers have followed these subjects into their elderly years so they could look back at their midlifes and see if they could predict who was going to grow into a happy, healthy octogenarian and who wasn't. And when they gathered together everything they knew about these subjects at age 50, it wasn't their midlife cholesterol levels or body mass indices that predicted how they were going to grow old. It was how satisfied they were in their relationships.

The people who were the most satisfied in their relationships at age 50 were the healthiest at age 80. The social support we get from our closest, most intimate relationships, it seems, not only offer some protection from the inevitable ups and downs of life, but may even mitigate the physical and emotional pains of aging. Academics call this "stress buffering."

According to the book, "Midlife is an inflection point, not only between young and old, but also between the self-focused, inward-looking way of living that many of us developed in young adulthood and a more generous, outward-looking way of living." In other words, just when our lives feel like they've narrowed in early midlife because we're juggling so much, this is the time to start focusing on how we invest in our relationships.

For many, midlife is when we start to treasure our relationships more than our possessions. And, as Dutch sociologist Gerald Mollenhorst has shown, we replace half of our social network every seven years or so, so investing in friendships is a lifelong endeavor. If you don't invest, your network will atrophy.

Laura Carstensen popularized the academic theory of socio-emotional selectivity, which states that younger people perceive time as more open-ended, and thus prioritize and pursue knowledge-related goals. In contrast, older individuals perceive time as more limited, and instead prioritize emotion-related goals. This is one more reason why midlife is the time to invest in your relationships. Social competition is replaced with social connectedness.

Relational Capital Is "Emotional Insurance"

Friends aren't a "nice-to-have." They're a "need-to-have."

The *Atlantic*'s Jennifer Senior suggests friends are the flora and fauna of our midlifes because we're so relentlessly busy. They become the wallpaper of our lives when, in fact, they're meant to be our comfy furniture, especially on a rainy day. What we forget is that some of our "furniture" has left town when a friend moves for a job or the friendship has been put in storage when family or work obligations become too much. Without investing in our friends, we may be left with an empty living room.

Myra Lavenue is a Portland-based lesbian, mother, writer, improv actor, and social justice advocate in her mid-50s. She's been with her wife for twenty-four years, and she has a large network of friends and work colleagues. Still, when I met her, she felt like a part of herself was closed off because of how busy she was and losses she'd had in her life.

When the pandemic hit the world, Myra was taking a beginning improv class. She'd joined the class because she felt adrift and bereft of community since retiring from recreational soccer, getting laid off from a company with a vibrant campus life, and becoming a fully remote worker at the new company she'd joined. As she sought clarity on how to cope with all these changes, a revelation for Myra was this: she needed to find her funny people. For her, humor is a form of spirituality. Could improv be the new place to find connection, friendship, *and* funny people?

Zoom might not be the ideal format for improv classes, but Myra recalls how it all began to click when "a woman joined a class I was taking, sitting quietly until her turn was called to be in a scene. And suddenly the screen was filled with her energy, presence, and focused talent. I was mesmerized, and sent a private Zoom message to her, saying 'You're funny!'"

Myra invited her new comic hero, Lisa, to an online storytelling class, then a musical improv class, and on to advanced improv classes. They exchanged numbers and the friendship sparks flew. A few months into their friendship, the COVID vaccines were released and they both got immunized. It was time to meet in person.

Myra bubbles over with emotion in telling me what happened next:

Bit by bit, we opened up our lives, homes, and families to each other. When she asked me if she could call me her best friend, I was so surprised because do adults talk like this? When was the last time I heard that question? Yet at the same time I felt my body receive that love in a huge rush of feeling that I shared with my wife.

Myra and Lisa are now "besties" who support each other's

creative endeavors, family issues, and—most importantly—personal growth and self-discovery. They're almost like the best friends we remember from grade school: making mischief, being too loud, not paying attention in class, and getting together for playdates. The key to how they got here was Lisa bravely stepping forward and asking that best friend question.

Who's a friend that you can get closer with? How might you see midlife as the time to be less self-conscious and more other-conscious? Are you willing to take the risk to say to someone, "I'd love to deepen our friendship. Are you open to that?"

Myra never realized, at age 56, how much she had been holding herself back from going deep with anyone other than her family. When you ask people who their best friends are, most will name the best friend they made in childhood, or maybe college. But best friends can be made at any age, and we must keep finding these connections, especially in midlife.

When we use the word *capital*, we often refer to wealth in the form of money or other assets owned by a person or organization. But relational capital is another form of wealth, the wealth we accrue from investing in relationships. You have property and liability insurance for your home or car, so where is your emotional insurance for friendships?

Is it true that you are the sum of the five people closest to you? You've probably come across this idea on Instagram or heard it from some sage onstage. It's often a motivational speaker trying to convince you that you'll be happier, better looking, or more successful if you junk the losers in your life. Yes, there's some research that supports this premise, but

I'd like to expand this thinking beyond the surface-level concerns. Let's reframe the question.

What if you knew that you were as deep or healthy or generous or empathetic or wise as the five people closest to you? Who are the people in your life that energize you or that you deeply admire? What is stopping you from spending more time with them?

How might you curate your friends as you do the flowers in your garden? How could you be good soil for those friendships?

I See You

We're living in the midst of a loneliness epidemic that was prevalent long before COVID. Much of the discussion around loneliness tends to center around kids and teens, but they aren't the only ones who are afflicted. According to a survey conducted in the spring of 2020 by the Roots of Loneliness Project, the demographic group that is experiencing the sharpest rise in loneliness in the United States is Gen X women (ages 41 to 57). And the increase in social isolation reported by women living with children was sharpest among those Gen Xers, according to an unpublished portion of the survey shared with the *Wall Street Journal*.

What most attempts to make sense of this trend overlook is the fact that in midlife, too many of us just don't feel seen. We feel invisible at work. Anonymous to our neighbors. A stranger to friends or family, who still see us as we were twenty years ago. To be invisible is to be disconnected. And with this phenomenon comes the growing number of tragic "deaths of despair" stories, especially in midlife.

What we need is a massive "I See You" public health campaign to keep people out of the ICU. This is an alternative form of Intensive Care in which you feel seen and appreciated for who you are. The friends we make when we are younger will likely see us as the person we were then. This can feel like an uncomfortable shoe that's a size or two too small. The good news is that, even if we're out of practice, making new friends in midlife isn't nearly as daunting as we tend to think. It's like riding a bike again, after a long break.

Here are four steps you can take to increase your social wellness and feel seen and connected:

1. **Ask yourself: Are you socially isolated, or are you lonely?** There's a difference. Many people prefer social isolation even as the greatest risk of the pandemic is behind us. Some appreciate the solitude it has given them. Being alone is different than being lonely, as the former may be a choice, and the latter often feels like a prison sentence. If you're lonely, make a list of five or ten people in your life who used to be friends. Then, stack rank them in terms of who you most would like to talk with and feel comfortable reaching out to. And then, once per week, reach out to one of those people to strike up a conversation and see how they're doing.

2. **Become adept at listening.** A wise person once said, "Knowledge speaks and wisdom listens." It's around

midlife that we appreciate that the people we love most aren't just interesting; they're also interested...in us, no less! To show that *you're* interested in the people *you* care about, try practicing Appreciative Inquiry: asking catalytic questions to unlock people's deepest thoughts, emotions, hopes, and dreams. Google it! It's a human form of A.I.

3. **No more "bowling alone."** When I was visiting my sons and their moms in Houston, we went to Ethan's Little League game, where I felt that kind of lovely community vibe of a tribe of parents coming together to support their kids. There was an older man there who I thought might be a grandpa. When I asked him which of the players he was related to, he said, "All of them. I've adopted the Pirates as my team." He was a widower, he told me, and lived down the street from a couple of the players and their parents. When he'd go on walks with his dog, he said, he'd walk by these kids' homes, hoping they would be playing in the front yard. The kids loved his dog, he explained, and eventually their parents had befriended him and invited him to a Little League game. "I'm teaching the whole team how to bowl," he added. The lesson? It's never too late to join a new community.

4. **Find your flock or build your own.** Birds of a feather flock together. You're more likely to forge new friendships with people who share your interests, and you can easily find these flocks in local Meetup or Facebook

groups. When I was going through a particularly challenging time and wanted deeper spiritual connections, I started hosting a Spiritual Sangha Dinner at my home once a month for a disparate collection of friends and acquaintances who followed quite different spiritual or religious paths. Pulling it off required a little courage and some social alchemy, but the magnetic topics we would discuss rounded off any sharp edges of our personalities and beliefs. Might you consider creating a book or film club, and building a new flock of your own?

What Can Be Learned from *The Velveteen Rabbit*?

Margery Williams's classic children's book, *The Velveteen Rabbit*, offers an insight that ought to be plastered on every midlifer's bathroom mirror, "Generally, by the time you are Real, most of your hair has been loved off."

As a nearly-bald guy in his early 60s, I can relate. Of course, with or without hair, it's easy to feel shabby and worn out as you get older. Fortunately, with receding hairlines and all the sagging bits and bobs of our aging body comes the perspective and the wisdom to know how beautiful life can be when we finally become the person we were meant to be all along and to celebrate that with others.

How wonderful it is to finally (at long last) venture into the timeless world of the heart and soul. After all, this is the natural progression of aging, which is perfectly captured in the full excerpt from *The Velveteen Rabbit*, the story of a stuffed rabbit's desire to become real through the love of his owner:

> You become. It takes a long time. That's why it doesn't often happen to people who break easily, or have sharp edges, or who have to be carefully kept. Generally, by the time you are Real, most of your hair has been loved off, and your eyes drop out and you get loose in the joints and very shabby. But these things don't matter at all, because once you are Real you can't be ugly, except to people who don't understand.

I say three cheers for the Velveteen Rabbit—our soft reminder that in midlife, it's time to get Real about who we are—and share that Real self with others. Let's get Real together!

5.

"I Have No More 'Fucks' Left to Give"

This may seem an incongruous chapter to follow my lovely ruminations on emotional intelligence and the value of relationships, but stay with me for a few pages. For many of you, this may be the most important chapter in this book.

Years ago, there was a pop psychology book that became the rage, *Don't Sweat the Small Stuff*. Replace "Small Stuff" with "Small-Minded People" and you have a hint of what's ahead for you in this chapter.

Earlier in my life, I found it hard to make decisions without getting others to weigh in. Whether I was playing a sport or writing an essay, I always wanted feedback (and, of course, approval) as if life was just one big performance. I'll never forget when I was elected student body president of our Long Beach Poly High School, one of my so-called friends, Jeanne, who fancied herself a rebellious artist, came up to me and said, "I don't like you." Taken aback, I asked why and she retorted, "Because everyone else likes you." Couldn't do much about that, could I?! But, despite it being a compliment, in its own weird way, it still seriously messed with my seventeen-year-old head.

Of course, it's never been easier to "sweat the small stuff" than it is today, thanks to Facebook and Instagram, with their endless likes, humblebrags, and preening, which have taken our tendency to package ourselves for others to a whole new level.

The good news is, there comes a time in our lives when we stop counting our "likes," wordsmithing our posts, and airbrushing our photos. As we age, most of us simply don't care what other people think in the same way we did before. We realize that "giving a fuck" is not only distracting, it drains our energy and our souls. In midlife, we begin to reclaim that energy for more important endeavors.

Survival of the Nicest?

This is not a new problem, Arthur Brooks reminds us, in an article for *The Atlantic*, appropriately titled "No One Cares!": As the Roman Stoic philosopher Marcus Aurelius wrote almost 2,000 years ago, "We all love ourselves more than other people, but care more about their opinion than our own."

Throughout human history, Brooks says, our survival has depended on the approval of others; we needed it to preserve our membership in close-knit clans and tribes, lest we be cast out from our group and sentenced to certain death from cold, starvation, or predators. This may be why physical pain and social rejection share the same neural substrates in our brain, he explains. It may also be why some of us live by the creed "survival of the nicest," even as we angrily grind our teeth in our sleep.

I'll admit it. I've spent my life as a people-pleaser. When I was young, I needed social validation because I felt like such an oddball. My parents considered sending me to pre-adolescence therapy because I preferred my imaginary friends to real ones; the friends I conjured were guaranteed to like me, and made for a captive audience. Eventually, this little introvert converted.

I became an admiration addict to protect myself from feeling inadequate. I had a scorecard in my head of just how much everyone in my life appreciated me. I was so damn savvy at this that I identified the three most popular boys in my junior high school—Alan, Erik, and Mike—and I devised a way to become their Fourth Musketeer! I gave a big fuck. That's for sure.

As a closeted jock in high school (and college) with loving girlfriends, the word "fuck" sent shivers down my spine, but, of course, in my college fraternity, it's all we talked about. My sex life became performative, both for my girlfriends, as well for my bros, to whom I recounted my sexual exploits. When I think back on all this, I feel suffocated and ashamed.

I came out as a gay man at 22, in the summer of 1983 while working in New York City. Once again, the big f-word was all we talked about in my new clan, and once again, sex became the currency with which to acquire the social approval I so craved.

Some people shed their people-pleasing instincts once they begin to achieve some career success, but as a baby CEO of the boutique hotel company I started when I was 26, I was extra sensitive to what people thought of me, partly because I was an unusual specimen—a very young, gay CEO in a traditionally stuffy industry in the 1980s—and partly because the hospitality business is all about making people happy. So giving a fuck has been baked inside me for a very long time.

Being a hotelier stretched my niceness to its extreme, until I realized just how self-obsessed many people are. This revelation—that most people are far too busy thinking about themselves to give a fuck about me—was what cured me. I started reading psychology books and learning personality-typing tools like the Enneagram to help me understand that I'm not the only weirdo out there.

I came to realize we all consistently overestimate how much other people think about us. I learned that because we focus on our own failings with laser-like intensity, we assume everyone else is doing the same: observing our blunders under a microscope (they aren't).

It's like when I learned how to surf in my 50s, near my home in Baja. I was sure all those folks sitting on the beach were watching me and only me flailing as a beginning surfer, even when there were a few dozen of us out there trying to catch waves. Naturally, my preoccupation with what I looked like created performance anxiety that got in the way of my ability to attune with the waves.

My solution was to try catching waves at dawn, when no one else was on the beach. And just like with yoga, once I got the hang of it, I came to realize that surfing—while an individual sport—is a fellowship, and that my solo surf sessions were depriving me of all the joy in hanging out with friends in the waves or on shore. That was when I finally stopped giving a fuck how I looked on the board.

Not Giving a Fuck Allows You to Give a Fuck

Mark Manson's book, *The Subtle Art of Not Giving a F*ck: A Counterintuitive Approach to Living a Good Life*, has sold more than 16 million copies since 2016. Clearly, we're not the only ones out there who've realized that the key to living a good life is not giving a damn about most things, but rather, caring quite a bit only about the things that matter.

Giving a fuck about less is particularly valuable in midlife, when we realize we've spent the first half of our life accumulating and now it's time for some editing. Learning how to prioritize the various elements of our lives is one of the most important endeavors as we age. As Belinda Mackie says in *The Good No*, Manson's point is "Not giving a fuck isn't about being indifferent. It's about feeling comfortable with being different."

Unfortunately, too much of the time, we're terrified about

what others think of us, partly because it may validate our most secret self-loathing. Look folks, by midlife, the only validation you need is for your parking.

Personally, I've learned to use my values as a filter for investing my time. There was a period in my life when I was asked to be on the board of directors for what felt like every damn nonprofit in San Francisco. At one time, I was on six boards that ranged from the arts to homelessness to children's education to preserving parkland to advocating for marriage equality to who knows what else. Yes, these were noble causes I wanted to support, but there was only so much Chip to go around! I came to realize that I gave the most serious hoot about urban poverty, so I joined the board of an inner-city church doing good work in a challenging neighborhood (I write more about this in chapter 12) and I phased out the rest of the boards.

You may have only a limited number of fucks to give over your lifetime, so you must spend them with care. As we hit midlife, we've developed a discernment for what truly matters. Our values define what activities have value. A wise person once said, "Your beliefs become your thoughts, your thoughts become your words, your words become your actions, your actions become your habits, your habits become your values, your values become your destiny."

Londoner Kay Scorah grew up in the north of England, where her paternal grandmother, a suffragette, trade union leader, and campaigner for equality, made her aware, through protests and activism, that the only way to leave the world a better place was to do something to fix what's wrong with it, not just talk about it. She taught Kay not to comply with the system, but to rebel or even to revolt.

Kay believed her grandmother, but, as is true for so many of us, her pragmatism intervened, and she ended up on a somewhat conventional career path, working in West Germany as a scientist. When she was in her 20s, she and her boyfriend feared that, if they were to succeed as scientists, they would have to leave behind the parts of them that wanted to change the world, to write poetry, to dance and make music. They called it "the cage," because they were afraid that the things that brought them joy would not bring them recognition—financial or societal—and dreaded being trapped by success.

Although Kay didn't stick with the biological sciences, that fear was realized. Trapped by a successful business career, by her ego, by financial necessity, but mainly by her own lack of self-belief, she lamented having left behind so much of herself. It was the gift of age that finally began to release her from her cage: from her race for more, her duty to support the family, and her desire to conform to society's definition of success.

So, in her late 40s and early 50s, she began to take a little time away from the paid work to make theater shows, write, take dance class and, most terrifying of all, try her hand at stand-up comedy. Now in her late 60s, she chooses to live in a tiny one-bedroom apartment, drives a small fifteen-year-old car inherited from her late father, has given away most of her possessions, and spends as much time as she can mentoring younger people because she often learns as much from them as they do from her. And she's never been happier.

She feels freed from the weight of those expectations society has of professional women: that she be not only harder working and more brilliant than her male counterparts, but also conform to society's expectations of female beauty. She rejected the values that society imposed on her without her permission, and now she says, "I am an invisible woman. What a relief!"

This sentiment has even made its way into her comedy routine:

Women my age complain about invisibility. Doesn't bother me at all; in fact, it's very useful in my work as a shoplifter and occasional assassin. I'm at that time of a woman's life that I call "Senopause." The place between the end of menopause and the beginning of senility. It's a very dangerous age where there is no nice lady hormone left.

Like most comedy acts, these jokes are grounded in reality. She believes that her invisibility, combined with her lack of visible wealth, allows her to confront and stand up to bullies and to call out bad behavior. She is no longer a threat or a target, so she can say what she likes. "Other people's assumptions of my frailty give me strength and courage," she explains. "I have nothing that anyone else wants except my wisdom and my opinions."

Kay is a great role model for not worrying about how you look or speak but, rather, how you act. And today, she's acting on her activism, working to bring about change not only for herself, but for the planet and her community.

Kay Scorah doesn't give many fucks anymore, but the ones she does give are deeply meaningful for her and others.

People Are Mirrors

We are all mirrors for each other. Kay's activism in her late 60s offers a role model to women as much as three generations younger. As we age, we sometimes forget just how much younger people long for us to shine the light on a healthier, happier path in our later years, since (if we're lucky) we're all traversing that path someday.

The much-loved Christian mystic Richard Rohr has written dozens of books and has a large global following made up of people of all ages, who deeply appreciate his universal, loving perspective on religion. As his neighbor in New Mexico, where MEA is creating two large campuses, we were honored that he chose to come to Baja in 2021 to experience MEA at age 78 as a student, not a teacher.

In his book *Falling Upward: A Spirituality for the Two Halves of Life*, Richard says,

Much of the work of midlife is learning to tell the difference between people who are still dealing with their issues through you and those who are really dealing with you as you really are.... By the second half of life, you learn to tell the difference between who you really are and how others can mirror that or not. This will keep you from taking either insults or praise too seriously.

He continues:

I doubt whether this kind of calm discrimination and detachment is much possible before your mid-50s at the earliest. How desperately we need true elders in our world to clean up our seeing and to stop the revolving hall of mirrors in its tracks.

To judge others is to judge oneself. If there's one lesson I've learned at this stage in my life, it's that welcoming equanimity into my heart is the number one way I can be good to myself. Developing a mental calmness, a composure, especially when I might be triggered by someone else, somehow relaxes my internal judgment toward myself. Tired of my buttons being pushed, I'm choosing my battles wisely.

Here are some of my favorite tips for not being triggered when I shouldn't give a flying fuck:

1. I ask myself, "Over the course of my lifetime, how important is this?"
2. I spend less time on social media and refuse to "doom-scroll."

3. I've stopped seeking a "permission slip" to do some-thing I care about.

4. I feel comfortable saying no to more of the things that have historically felt obligatory.

I also regularly recite these three sentences, which Stephen Covey felt expressed the wisdom of Holocaust survivor Vik-tor Frankl: "Between stimulus and response, there is a space. In that space is our power to choose our response. In our response lies our growth and our freedom."

I find that space by taking regular "awe walks" with my dog Jamie. I schedule these walks in my calendar under the title "spying on the divine." An awe walk is particularly valu-able for those in midlife and beyond, not just for the exercise, but because it helps us to feel the presence of something larger than us. Something mysterious, ineffable, and beautiful. I try to do these walks in new locations as often as I can, as I'm more likely to experience the childlike wonder of seeing something new.

It's hard to hold on to the toxic energy we feel after being triggered by a person in our life when we're marveling at an industrious hummingbird or seeing a tangle of vines climb-ing an oak tree. Awe is all about getting outside the cage of our ego and recognizing that we can be a "first-class noticer" of something beyond our frustrating friend or our annoying neighbor. Before I embark upon an awe walk, I always ask the question, "Nature, what do you have to teach me today?"

What if nature could be your mirror?

You Are Only as Big as the Problems That Annoy You

The word *annoy* has an illuminating etymology based on the Latin *in odio*, "It is hateful to me." We all feel hateful on occasion, especially in our increasingly polarizing sociopolitical world. But let's be judicious about the hate bombs; after all, you are the container for that toxic substance and, no doubt, it can be internally corrosive.

Everyone has their triggers. But in midlife, we realize we can be more discerning about what bothers the shit out of us. We can let most things roll off our backs, and save our mental and emotional energy for the few things that deserve our vigilant attention. As one of my activist friends says, "The longer I stay on the planet, the noisier I will get. But I'm more selective about when I make that noise."

Or, when you start to feel triggered, you could just take some advice from comedian Ricky Gervais: "Be happy. It really annoys negative people." But don't do it to annoy people, as that would be giving a fuck. I recently saw this on a T-shirt of someone who was maybe twenty years my senior: "A wise woman once said fuck this shit and she lived happily ever after." I gave this woman I didn't know a big hug.

THE MENTAL
LIFE

6.

"I'm Marveling at My Wisdom"

Knowledge is in your phone.
Wisdom is in your gut.

Generally, midlifers get a bad rap when it comes to their mental capacity. Not only are we perceived as being hopeless with technology, it's also around this time that people start making jokes about our memory or comprehension speed.

This section of the book is not about how to ensure that your mind doesn't trail your life span or health span. Don't worry, I'm not thrusting any sudoku puzzles at you. This is about why you should rest assured that these assumptions about the middle-aged brain are largely unfounded (for one thing, some of the most brilliant technologists I know are in their 50s and 60s): that in fact, some mental competencies actually *improve* with age.

Yes, our ability to process new information, learn, and solve problems—what's known as fluid intelligence—is at its peak in our early 20s. And most of us probably wouldn't fare as well on SATs as we did when we took the test thirty or more years ago.

On the other hand, as Arthur C. Brooks documents in his bestselling book, *From Strength to Strength*, our brain's ability to think holistically—what's known as crystallized intelligence—improves with age. In fact, our crystallized intelligence doesn't peak until age 70.

Moreover, the longer we've been on the planet, the more knowledge and experience we've accumulated, and the more patterns we've seen. These are the raw materials for wisdom. By midlife, we're experts in the school of life. We've become masters at pattern recognition. We can connect the dots faster, and more effectively.

After all, as Steve Jobs suggested in his Stanford commencement address nearly two decades ago, "You can't connect the dots looking forward; you can only connect them looking backward." The longer you've lived, the more "backward" you have.

As we get older, we also get more adept at moving between the left brain and the right brain; this is how we can be both logical and lyrical in the same sentence. It's also part of the reason we become alchemists as we age. I don't know about you, but my ability to synthesize seemingly opposite qualities is at its peak. Curiosity and wisdom. Yin and yang. Extrovert and introvert. Secular and spiritual. Doing and being. Mentor and intern. Gravitas and levity. My intuition about which of these two polarities are needed at any particular moment feels like magic.

Then there is wisdom. Wisdom is correlated with crystallized intelligence, but there's more to it than that. Dr. Dilip Jeste highlights seven components of wisdom:

- An ability to self-reflect
- A strong skill in emotional regulation
- An acceptance of diverse perspectives
- Prosocial behaviors and aptitude (empathy, compassion, altruism)
- Decisiveness
- An ability and desire to socially advise (give helpful advice to others)
- An interest in spirituality and finding deeper meaning in life

How many of these components have been growing stronger in you as you've entered midlife?

The Man Who Mistook His Knowledge for Wisdom

You know the guy I'm talking about. He's the brainiac, the walking encyclopedia who constantly recites arcane facts but has zero self-awareness and appears to have no idea what "mansplaining" means. He's the one who knows Albert

Einstein's birthday but forgets his own wedding anniversary. He understands nuclear physics but is hopeless when it comes to understanding humans. He's the "knowledge worker" who desperately could use a "wisdom worker" by his side.

At a time when we're awash in knowledge, where is the wisdom the world so desperately needs?

Knowledge is "local." Wisdom, however, is "global" — and portable; it can take you places you never imagined, well outside your usual sphere of influence and expertise. Yes, knowledge may be power, but wisdom is wealth, mentally and spiritually. Knowledge is static, and risks obsolescence with time. Meanwhile, wisdom becomes more potent in your life the longer it ferments. Knowledge is simple interest. Wisdom is compounding interest.

Your wisdom has your fingerprints all over it. It can't be found in an encyclopedia. It is based upon your unique experiences, history, insight, and humanity. It can't be replicated.

Skills are to knowledge what practices are to wisdom. In this chapter, I'll offer you a few wisdom practices that you can incorporate into your life.

Philosopher and psychologist John Dewey writes, "Information is knowledge which is merely acquired and stored up; wisdom is knowledge operating in the direction of powers to the better living of life." As we venture deeper into midlife and the file cabinet in our brain begins to feel fuller and fuller, being able to discern the essential from the tangential is an increasingly valuable skill.

I used to define wisdom as purely "metabolized experience," but that now feels incomplete. So my new definition of wisdom is "metabolized experience that leads to distilled compassion." A savvy person metabolizes their experience, but a wise person imparts the resulting insights for the common good. I call it "distilled compassion" because a wise person offers compassion in a way that is uniquely tailored to the person receiving it.

One of the revelations I've experienced since starting the Modern Elder Academy is how many young people are motivated to cultivate and harvest their wisdom. Who would have guessed that more than 15 percent of the people coming to a program with *Elder* in its name would be Millennials?

At 39, Adam McCants is one Millennial who has assiduously cultivated a relationship with wisdom early in his midlife. He is a faithful journeyer who had experienced the loss of multiple loved ones by the time he was a young adult. He believes those losses accelerated the growth of his own wisdom and compassion. Passionate about communicating hope to others, and motivated to apply his curiosity and knack for technology to the mental health space, Adam is creating tools that allow people to better process what they're going through emotionally.

For Adam, wisdom breeds empathy. Knowledge is objective, neutral, and emotionless, but wisdom has a heart. Cultivating his wisdom at a young age has influenced Adam's career direction and probably saved him from the typical midlife career crisis many people experience.

As author David Brooks says,

Out of your own moments of suffering comes a compassionate regard for the frailty of others.... Wise people don't tell us what to do, they start by witnessing our story. They take the anecdotes, rationalizations and episodes we tell, and see us in a noble struggle. They see our narratives both from the inside, as we experience them, and from the outside, as we can't.

At 41 and with two young sons, a growing business, aging parents, and increasing financial and political influence, Caleb Quaid started witnessing his own story. Like Adam and many other Millennials, Caleb has been on a fast track since early adulthood. As the Director of Business Administration and Project Director for the Tampa Bay Buccaneers in the National Football League, he oversaw more than $200 million in capital projects for the Bucs, where he spent a decade. The job created huge sacrifices in his work-life balance, especially as a young father.

Even after the team, led by Tom Brady (truly a modern elder of the NFL), won the Super Bowl and Caleb earned a Super Bowl ring with his name etched on it, he felt a hollowness inside. His internal wisdom told him that his passion was no longer football, but he was instead to become an entrepreneur in the burgeoning "regeneration" world. Ironically, one of his new clients for his firm Regenerative Shift is his former employer, the Buccaneers. He's planted a 1,100-square-foot living fence of bamboo and native plants at Raymond James Stadium. Caleb credits his investment in seeking wisdom through Buddhist principles with finding a better life so that he might avert a crisis in his late 40s.

There are three generations that can claim they're in midlife these days—Boomers, Gen Xers, and Millennials. I'm encouraged that Millennials might finally help us rebrand midlife as an age dedicated to our calling, not a crisis.

How I Started Harvesting Wisdom at Age 28

"No one was ever wise by chance." These words tumbled out of the Stoic philosopher Seneca's mouth more than 2,000 years ago. Today, they're an important reminder that pursuing wisdom is a choice, and it's often the result of a skinned knee or a bruised ego. In other words, our current difficulties create our future gifts.

At age 28, I was struggling as the young CEO of my boutique hotel company. The 1989 earthquake had rocked San Francisco, leaving parts of the city on fire, the Bay Bridge collapsed, and many San Franciscans hunkered down in their homes. No one knew how long the aftershocks would continue and, for the next six months, my one and only hotel was operating at less than half of its normal occupancy. I was running out of cash and didn't know what to do.

A friend of mine suggested I start writing in a diary, maybe because he was tired of hearing me kvetch. As I limped into one particular weekend, I took down an empty diary from my bookshelves and stared at it for a few minutes, hoping it would do the writing for me. I loudly played "We Are the Champions" on an endless loop because that same friend told me it's what got him out of a bad mood. Didn't work for me... or my neighbors.

When it became clear that the pages of this diary would not fill themselves, I started writing down what I'd learned that week: lessons from the school of hard knocks. These bullet-point lessons read almost like tips one might give to a loved one. That loved one was me.

For example, one was a lesson I'd learned when I went to my banker that week and asked if I could take out a line of credit. He told me I should have made the request pre-earthquake, and quickly taught me the first rule of lending: never lend to someone who needs it, only to those who don't really need the cash. Dude, if I had that kind of magical foresight, I wouldn't be managing a hotel in a dodgy part of San Francisco!

Another was a lesson about enlisting natural-born skeptics to support a new idea before presenting it to a leadership team. That week, I had what I thought was a brilliant, if a bit outlandish, marketing idea: to attract Northern California residents, we would rent a snow machine and park it in our hotel's poolside courtyard so people could make snowmen when they came to San Francisco to do their holiday shopping. Just as quickly as I unleashed this idea on my team, a couple of the skeptics unleashed all the reasons it wouldn't work, and the idea melted faster than a California snowman. If I'd met one-on-one with both of the skeptics before the meeting and gotten their feedback on how this idea could be improved, maybe they would have been more supportive in the team meeting.

After thirty minutes of reflecting on my week, I hand-wrote "My Wisdom Book" on the cover, and a tradition was hatched. Each weekend, I would dutifully record some of my biggest lessons of the past week (mainly relating to my career or leadership, but also in my personal life), and what I had learned from them. Many decades later, I realized that this weekend ritual was a way for me to harvest and metabolize my wisdom to serve me and others in the future.

You can do the same. *This coming weekend, pull out an unused journal and jot down a few sentences about three or four different circumstances you encountered during the week, including how you handled them (even if you made a mistake or two) and what you learned from them. This is a practice that can accelerate the growth of your wisdom.*

Learning to Own Our Wisdom

In modern life, talking about wisdom can feel taboo, even though it's been discussed for thousands of years. Perhaps that's because while knowledge is obvious, wisdom is more ephemeral, maybe even mystical. As David Brooks indicates in his essay "Wisdom Isn't What You Think It Is," popular examples of the wise sage — he lists Yoda, Dumbledore, and Solomon — are hard to relate to. And, of course, anyone who proclaims loudly that they're wise is a bit of an embarrassment. That's the wisdom conundrum: no wise person professes to be wise.

By midlife, it's time to start owning up to the fact that, assuming a certain amount of intentionality, you've developed some wisdom over your years. Think of wisdom as the crossroads where the pragmatics of life meet the psychology of humans. You can be the crossing guard at this intersection. How well do you understand yourself and your fellow members of this species?

In Brooks's essay, he writes that wise people "are more like story editors than sages." When you look at it that way, wisdom suddenly seems far more accessible. You don't need to be some white-robed wizard dispensing the secrets of life, or some motivational speaker spouting million-dollar clichés. You can be a "motivational listener," someone who is so attuned at becoming a first-class noticer that you see the through line narrative in your best friend's sobbing story. You are a compassionate prober, which means that your questions aren't meant to serve you and show how smart you are; they're meant to serve others. It means you offer fresh eyes, and a wise soul.

In our younger years, many of us are overtrained in analysis and undertrained in perception (thanks to Peter Drucker for that insight). We know how to think, but we haven't sufficiently learned how to *see and feel*. Most of us glance at the world, but we don't see what's beneath the surface. But in midlife, we become mindful and patient enough to look deeper, long enough for our pattern-recognizing intuition to kick in. Live in that place of wisdom, and your presence will genuinely become a present to those who surround you.

By midlife, you can see around corners. You've developed the peripheral vision required to see the potential collateral upside and downside of a decision. And you've learned to recognize your blind spots and avoid falling into old patterns. If only you'd honed these abilities in your 20s when you took that big-bucks job that jaded your soul, or married the wrong spouse because of what everyone else thought about her.

Ask yourself, "Do I trust my decision making today more than I did twenty years ago?" If your answer is yes, why don't you take a little more pride in the wisdom you've developed?

How Can I Get (Even) Wiser?

Wisdom is a limitless resource we can develop more of at any age, as the raw material of wisdom, our life experience, is a 24/7/365 endeavor. But it doesn't happen without intention. Here are a few ways to actively and intentionally develop your wisdom as an essential life skill.

1. **Divulge your wisdom.** Every year, make a list of the five pieces of wisdom you might offer someone younger than you. The capital of Paraguay or how to make a martini won't be on your list. Your knowledge is not

your wisdom. You'll know it's original wisdom because it will come from your heart or gut, or the core of who you are. Consider doing this with a few friends and sharing your wisdom with one another.

2. **Recite the Serenity Prayer as a daily practice.** This is especially valuable when you're faced with challenging situations: "Grant me the serenity to accept the things I cannot change, the courage to change the things I can, and the wisdom to know the difference." Distinguishing between constants (things you can't change) and variables (things you can) doesn't just make you a mathematician; it makes you a wise human. This prayer is valuable whether you're religious or not.

3. **Counsel yourself in the third person.** We tend to have no trouble giving wise advice to someone else, but find it much harder to apply objectivity to ourselves. When a situation concerns you personally, advises Igor Grossman of the University of Chicago Wisdom Center, imagine that you are speaking to a distant or future self. Grossman suggests using third-person language ("What does Chip think?" instead of "What do I think?" or asking yourself "How will I respond a year from now?"), citing research showing "that such distancing strategies help people reflect on a range of challenges in a wiser, more objective fashion."

4. **Develop your intuition.** While there's been very little research on the connection between intuition and wisdom, both rely on crystallized intelligence and pattern

recognition. Create an intuition diary and keep it on your bedside table where you can record your dreams before they drift from memory; your subconscious is fertile ground for intuition. When you have an intuition about the character of a person, the outcome of a big career or financial decision, or even where you might experience a transformative vacation, write down the thought and the date. And, over time, see how many of your notions turn out to be true. You might start feeling more and more confident about your intuition.

5. **As a team, group, or family, make a practice of regularly asking yourself what you've learned.** As you now know, my Wisdom Book is one of my prized possessions. In the past, I've asked some of my leadership teams to dedicate a full in-person meeting to talking about what we've learned in the past quarter or year, and creating a record of our collective wisdom. This can be a means of both sharing insights and learning that expressing vulnerability (the opposite of being a know-it-all) can create deeper connections.

One of the greatest rewards of aging is seeing the seedlings of wisdom, planted in our younger years, growing healthy and strong inside ourselves. And what a treasure it is to share this wisdom with others. Just remember war stories aren't necessarily wisdom. Your history—if not metabolized, made fresh for the context of the situation, and offered humbly—might just earn you an "OK, Boomer" from someone younger.

As artificial intelligence continues to pervade our society and knowledge becomes more commodified, we're moving out of the information age into the intuition age. So watch out, robots, there's an army of midlifers ready, willing, and able to share their metabolized experience in a way that makes the world a better place.

7.

"I Understand How My Story Serves Me"

No one knows your life story better than you.

A novel is a good metaphor for the journey of life. When you're 25 years old, it's hard to think of your life as a coherent narrative. When you're a quarter of the way through a book, you really aren't sure where it's going, and if someone asked you what it was about, you might find it challenging to give an answer. But, by the time you're halfway through a novel, you know what it's about and can describe the themes, even if you don't know how it will end or what twists lie in store. Similarly, by the time you're 50, you've seen enough plot points to start seeing the through line.

In midlife, you can start becoming the enlightened witness to and screenwriter of this story. When we infuse our storytelling with our self-awareness, who knows what kind of masterpiece we might curate? This dense chapter—which could even be its own book (so feel free to read it twice)—will help you craft your masterpiece out of the raw material of your story.

Author Joseph Campbell, who popularized the idea of the Hero's Journey, believed in the discovery of truth through stories. In *The Hero with a Thousand Faces*, he describes the journey thus: "A hero ventures forth from the world of common day into a region of supernatural wonder: fabulous forces are there encountered and a decisive victory is won: the hero comes back from this mysterious adventure with the power to bestow boons on his fellow man."

Campbell ascribes three stages to this cyclical journey, as depicted in the diagram below: departure (separation), when the hero is compelled to leave the ordinary world; initiation, when the hero crosses into the other world and faces obstacles; and return, when the hero crosses the threshold back into the world from whence they came, which looks and feels different now, because the hero has changed.

One of the benefits of growing older is seeing the patterns or themes of our life. This isn't always pretty—but it is always revealing. Psychologist Carl Jung is famous for formulating the concept of the shadow, the portion of our personality which, through the course of our life, is relegated to the darkness of the unconscious. In his work *Aion*, he discusses the role of the unconscious in our lives. Some have paraphrased Jung thus: "That which we do not bring to consciousness appears in our lives as fate."

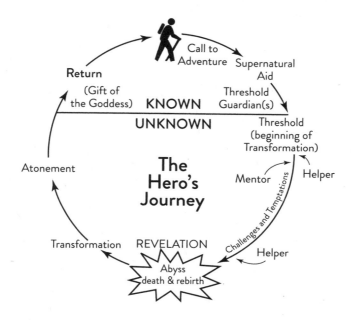

When I hear the word *fate*, I think of myths or stories shared huddled around a campfire, but fate isn't necessarily predestined. It's something we can influence if we're awake enough to see our patterns and modify our story.

Recently, I was introduced to Hollywood screenwriter Christopher Vogler's take on the Hero's Journey, one that may be familiar to those who watch a lot of movies. His twelve stages, listed below, inspired me to imagine my life as a Hero's Journey.

1. The Ordinary World
2. The Call to Adventure

3. Refusal of the Call
4. Meeting the Mentor
5. Crossing the First Threshold
6. Tests, Allies, and Enemies
7. Approach to the Inmost Cave
8. Ordeal, Death, and Rebirth
9. Reward (Seizing the Sword)
10. The Road Back
11. Resurrection
12. Return with Elixir

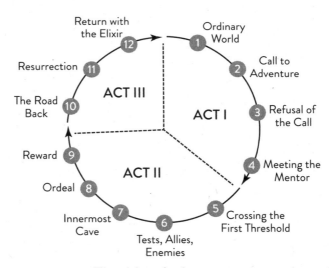

The Hero's Journey
Christopher Vogler's take on the monomyth

Source: Christopher Vogler, *The Writer's Journey* (Studio City, CA: 1998, Michael Wiese Productions).

As you'll see later in this chapter when I introduce you to Joelle Calton, this model can work for the hero or heroine because, at the end of the day, this isn't about being a hero, it's about being human.

My Hero's Journey

Usually sometime around midlife, we come to a point where we've seen enough of our own tricks and we come to feel that *my shadow self is who I am.* We face ourselves in our raw, unvarnished, and uncivilized state. This is the shadowland where we are led by our own stupidity, our own sin, our own selfishness, by living out of our false self. We have to work our way through this with brutal honesty, confessions and surrenders, some forgiveness, and often by some necessary restitution or apology. The old language would have called it repentance, penance, or stripping.

—*Richard Rohr,* The Art of Letting Go

The second half of my adult life has been my time to map out the emotional maze that has guided my thinking and actions. I've tried to be fearless and awake enough to see all my shadows, those personality traits—selfishness, impatience, pride—that lurk in the darkness.

For many, coming face-to-face with our shadow in midlife has us running for the hills. We're scared of something lurking below the surface of our life. We feel like we're a ventrilo-quist's dummy, but we don't realize we're the ventriloquist.

Your shadow isn't a flaw. It's a natural part of you. We all have one. Learning to see your shadow or the patterns that don't serve you requires a growth mindset, a willingness to improve even if it's occasionally painful to see your habits or beliefs in the magnifying mirror. Later in the chapter, we'll let you unleash your curiosity and sense of discovery on your shadow. But, for now, I'll take you on a midlife midnight stroll to my dark side and back.

During a recent holiday season, I did a vibrational heal-ing session with a South American shaman who used every-thing from sacred bells to a didgeridoo to awaken me from my year-end slumber (yes, I'm open to weird modalities to find insights). If you've ever done a "sound bath," you know this experience can calm your nervous system while shaking up your sense of reality. God knows, in midlife, we could use a little bit of shaking up of our "same old, same old" default ways of living.

The night after that session, I had vivid dreams. I saw myself as part Luke Skywalker (*Star Wars*) and part Neo (*The Matrix*) as I traversed what felt like a gauntlet of challenges. I'm not sure I have ever experienced a deeper sleep. In the morning, I felt compelled to write some notes to myself, and in the next twenty-four hours, my personal Hero's Journey emerged: the pattern I can see in so many of my endeavors in the course of my life.

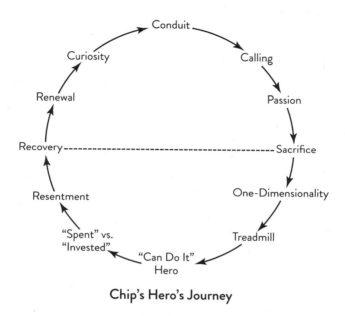

Chip's Hero's Journey

My starting point is the "Conduit" at the top of the circle. This is my default setting when life is good: to be a conduit of catalytic ideas. Whether it's my writing, my business ideas, or my intuition about people, when I'm at my best, I have an ability to tap into the zeitgeist to the point people call me a "zeitgeist surfer." At least that's one form of surfing I can do well! Having created this diagram, I now know that I need to better understand what conditions allow me to be the best conduit.

1. **Calling:** When my channel is open, my connection to the collective consciousness is five bars full of spiritual

Wi-Fi. It is in those times that I often feel called by an idea or premonition. My problem isn't picking up the call. It's occasionally having too many calls coming in at the same time and trying to distinguish which ones to focus my love and attention on. I'm Lily Tomlin's Ernestine character, the wry switchboard operator.

2. **Passion:** Once I answer the call, the raw potential of the idea stirs a passion in me, an energy to engage with this calling even if it wakes me up out of my comfortable world. I love it when I feel this current flowing through my veins, especially now, in midlife, an era that many consider a time of dormancy.

3. **Sacrifice:** The natural outgrowth of passion is a willingness to sacrifice. This is where the liminal stage of the Hero's Journey begins. In the modern world, making a sacrifice sounds like self-inflicted suffering or loss, but I see it as synonymous with devotion, an opportunity to pledge my loyalty and enthusiasm to something bigger than myself.

4. **One-Dimensional Focus:** This is where I drop below the surface of what's familiar, and things can start getting dicey. My habitual tendency is to become so focused on this new passion that I can neglect other parts of my life. This is when I start hearing (and trying to drown out) the voices of friends and family who wonder if I've lost my marbles. But, at this stage of the journey, I feel like I've found my midlife marbles.

5. **Treadmill:** Then, because I'm a bit of an achievement addict, I tend to jump on the treadmill and start running toward this calling. My ambition kicks in, and I keep turning up the speed. I'm a classic entrepreneur: I don't know my limits until I've surpassed them. I live by the spirit of the children's book *The Little Engine That Could*: "I think I can, I think I can, I think I can..."

6. **"Can Do It" Hero:** At the bottom of this cycle, my rugged individualist ego emerges big time. For those of you who know the three on the Enneagram, this is me, fully amped, like a locomotive. The problem with this point in my journey can be summed up by the adage, "If you want to go fast, go alone. If you want to go far, go together." I can start being out of sync with my team. I have an existential impatience with everyone, including myself.

7. **"Spent" vs. "Invested":** When I'm living my calling and feeling my purpose, I have intense stamina and a high threshold for pain—that is, until I hit the occasional wall and realize how exhausted I am. That's when I wonder whether I'm "spent" or "invested" with respect to this endeavor. I always hope that I'm invested, but on a bad day, I feel spent. And it's in those spent moments that I hit my nadir, found at point eight on this journey.

8. **Resentment:** This is when the resentment can start seeping in. Why am I the one having to do this, that, or the other? Why can't others keep up with me or do

more? This is when I become the victim, a role I loathe in myself and others. You've heard of "Mercury in retrograde," right? This is my "circuitry in retrograde." This is me at my worst.

9. **Recovery:** Assuming I'm self-aware enough to know what's going on (or coworkers or friends clue me in), I look for ways to recover my sense of energy and intention, often by retreating from others and doing things that bring me back to life—physically, emotionally, and spiritually. I take awe walks (mentioned in chapter 6) and ramp up my meditation practice.

10. **Renewal:** Hopefully, at this stage, I'm seeing the fruits of all the labor. Even if I'm not returning home triumphant, I feel that I'm coming back a changed man, with all the new wisdom I've accumulated in process and the hope that I will be even wiser on my next adventure. This is a perfect time to reflect on my adventure and metabolize my experience.

11. **Curiosity:** Finally, I have the time and space to be curious, and the whole miraculous process can start again. Long ago, explorers went searching for the fountain of youth, but what I seek is the fountain of curiosity, as that's always the wellspring of my creativity and joy.

12. **"Conduit":** From "Conduit" to "Can do it" to "Conduit" over and over. This is a common pattern in my life. When I shift from "can do it" to "conduit," I don't feel like I'm working anymore. I'm flowing. I am the "conducted," not the conductor.

Until I was able to plot my story like this, I didn't quite understand how often I lived this pattern and how much my shadow lurked underneath the surface. I now see that this is a miraculous journey that I've felt guided on multiple times in my life. And, now that I have uncovered some of the shadow parts of my Hero's Journey, I hope that I can make the next journey feel less treacherous.

You may notice that my twelve stages on this journey don't match Christopher Vogler's from earlier in the chapter. Indeed, we each have to chart our own Hero's Journey; there are no formulas, only guides. And this Hero's Journey isn't a one-and-done proposition. And it doesn't define my whole life's journey; it's a journey I've traveled many times throughout my life.

I'm sure your Hero's Journey will look different than mine. It might have just six or eight stages, or it might have twenty, but in any such journey, there will be stages that seem in conflict. Once you've mapped out your own journey, draw a line between each stage and the one standing opposite, and take note of the polarity.

For me, Passion is opposite Resentment and One-Dimensional Focus is opposite holistic Renewal. Understanding these polarities tells us what's needed to bring us back into balance. In my case: to seek out more collaboration, to be careful with my tendency toward myopic thinking and laser-like focus when I dive into a passion project, and to incorporate wellness practices that restore me, especially when I'm most obsessed with a project.

The Hero's Journey is a life script that we are constantly revising.

What If You Imagined Your Life as a Hero's Journey?

Don't feel performance anxiety about conjuring up your Hero's Journey story. If you are struggling, think of it as a crossword puzzle and use the clues in your life to fill in the missing stages of your cyclical quest. Remember, in midlife you've experienced enough life to see a few patterns. To try this for yourself, consider the following guidance and questions:

1. **Start by imagining a pivotal time in your life that fits the three-part structure:** (a) departure from your normal life, (b) an initiation into an unknown world full of adventure or challenge, and (c) the return to what seems like your normal life, but changed because you have changed. It could be when you studied overseas in college, when you joined the military, or when you got married, for example. Some of these may have included a ceremony to mark your rite of passage: perhaps you attended an orientation, an initiation, or had a wedding. Think of the stage at the very top of the circle as your default position; the part of yourself that often acts as a catalyst for what's coming next: it could be your gut instinct, boredom, self-knowledge—or virtually anything else. For me, it is being the conduit for ideas.

2. **Don't feel like you need to draw a circle and fill it in at this early stage.** You don't have to list your stages in

order right out of the gate; just jot down whatever ideas come up. If you're drawing a blank, take another look at Christopher Vogler's twelve stages, mentioned earlier in this chapter. This might illuminate some of the key elements of your journey. Also, consider if there are any archetypes that define you—the magician, the caretaker, the explorer—that might influence how you articulate your journey.

3. **Identify the shadow parts of yourself that arose when you were outside your comfort zone.** As you embarked upon this journey, what were some of your emotions you felt when you encountered your first challenges, and how did you surmount them? Just know that the middle section of this journey was likely painful or at least adventurous, and may have brought you face-to-face with some part of your shadow personality (in my case, that meant overworking and feeling resentful). Then ask yourself how you felt when you came out on the other side. Did you feel a sense of accomplishment? An evolution in how you saw yourself and the world? If you're still feeling stuck, try writing a children's fairy tale of your life. Start with "Once upon a time…" and do your best to be objective and honest. You may be surprised by what epiphany emerges.

4. **Identify common frustrations, and work backward.** Try to come up with at least two or three seminal experiences in your life. Then take a step back and ask yourself, "What can I learn from my past patterns?" When

we feel we haven't learned something from past experiences, we tend to feel frustrated with ourselves. Work backward from that frustration. What shadow or emotion may have triggered you into this pattern? Was it envy, fear, risk-seeking, perfectionism, or one of the archetypal ways of being like the rebel who has to be different or the jester who uses jokes to deflect and distract?

5. **Draw a circle and lay out the stages of your story in what feels like the natural progression of your story.** You may find, as I did, that there are some polarities on opposite ends of the circle. And, now, ask yourself how might you use this drawing to help you understand your path moving forward.

Joseph Campbell says, "The first problem of the returning hero is to accept as real, after an experience of the soul-satisfying vision of fulfillment, the passing joys and sorrows, banalities and noisy obscenities of life." This is part of the reason that thrill-seekers often go out on another adventure soon after they've come home. They love the adrenaline rush of being out there in the world slaying dragons.

But, in your Hero's Journey, the dragon may slay YOU. If you are wise, you will be humbled and will learn. You'll dust yourself off and live by the Japanese saying, "Fall down seven times, get up eight." You don't have to win. You just have to savor the victory of becoming wiser as a result of this journey. If you don't, you may find yourself playing the same movie over and over again, complaining about the new job or boss or spouse after you've jilted the old ones. A "change" is circumstantial and situational, but a true "transition" is psychological and spiritual.

Your Hero's Journey should make an indelible mark on your mind and soul so you are forever changed. And reflecting on your journey will give you a clear road map for how you curate the second half of your adulthood more consciously and joyfully.

Joelle's Hero's Journey

Joelle Calton was born into a small town of five hundred people in the Sacramento–San Joaquin River Delta, a longtime agricultural community with not much more than a general store and a bar on Main Street. Over the decades, the town spoiled its residents with a bounty of cherries and peaches as it crippled them with poverty and lack of opportunity. Joelle and her mother were incredibly poor and lived in basements, in single-wide trailers, and in migrant housing for much of her childhood.

Meanwhile, her father's life in San Francisco seemed rich and shiny, due to his successful rise in real estate after overcoming his own childhood poverty in southern Missouri. As the father of four, he made it his mission to expose his children to as many experiences and opportunities as he could, especially educational support. But, early in her life, Joelle's parents got divorced. Being the youngest child, Joelle was separated from her siblings, who went to live with her father while she remained in her small town with mom. Though she wasn't consciously aware of it at the time, this was when Joelle first realized that she needed to be self-sufficient and practical in order to survive.

Joelle says, "My hero's journey isn't one of sudden, dramatic turns. I didn't get whisked out of Kansas by a tornado. No one handed me a ring or light saber to bear, culminating in a final battle for salvation and purpose. No single burning passion drove me toward good choices and away from bad ones."

Her journey was slow and winding. Plagued by self-doubt and a perceived lack of options, she dropped out of high school. She started and stopped college four times. And she waited tables for fifteen years before eventually graduating, finishing her second doctorate program, and launching a career as a practicing psychologist.

Looking back, it was an invitation from an unlikely mentor—her father, who came back into her life when she was an adult—that finally gave her permission to launch. And maybe that's all any of us need: someone to see us, reflecting back at us that which we can't see, offering a subtle invitation to stretch, to pursue something unfamiliar, to grow. But it rarely happens in a single life-altering AHA! moment. There may be a moment that moves us from intention to action, but as a culmination of the thousands of little moments that came before.

As Joelle puts it, "They say there is death by a thousand cuts, but perhaps there is growth by a thousand cuts as well."

Joelle continues,

> I saw that through all the twists and turns, through two careers that couldn't seem more different on the sur-face, I leaned on the same skills to guide me through my early and later life: meeting people where they are, anticipating their needs due to my intuition, and feel-ing honored and humbled to be brought into their expe-rience, attunement, and discernment. And although I hung up my restaurant server's apron at 31 and will hang up my practicing psychologist's shingle at 56, I know that those same skills will be—MUST be—an integral part of wherever my journey takes me next.

At midlife, Joelle finally feels like she's started to see the bigger picture. Being a server isn't all that different from being a shrink, she has come to realize. After all, whether celebrat-ing an anniversary or going through a difficult divorce, people need to be cared for, seen, and met where they are. Now mar-ried for the first time at age 56 and a (step)mother for the first time, she's applying those same skills in her new role.

Today, she feels more self-sufficient, more confident, than her childhood self ever dreamed was possible, thanks to the knowledge that she's developed some wisdom—and some portable skills—along the way.

The deep understanding of people that Joelle developed early in life has been a through line in her story. While she struggled with school (what she calls her "ordeal," using Christopher Vogler's model), she's always had a natural curiosity about people and the world. And her life experiences required her to build self-reliance and resilience, which meant she often carried a rebellious spirit about her as she heeded her "call to adventure."

This, in turn, helped her to learn more about herself and develop a discernment and wisdom that allowed her to serve others. And, as an extrovert, she is fueled by the sense of

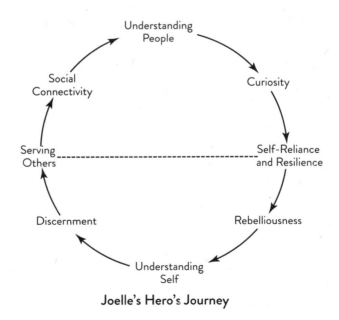

Joelle's Hero's Journey

connection she derives from serving other people and by her deep relationships with a close set of friends—which takes her back to the top of the circle again.

As you can see, as is true with my Hero's Journey, the juxtapositions are quite illuminating. Understanding People opposite Understanding Self. Self-Reliance & Resilience opposite Serving Others.

The Agency to Write Our Own Script

We have a choice in how we tell our life story. We don't write it in permanent ink. There are no points for consistency, or even accuracy. We can change it at any time, for any reason, including one as simple as making ourselves feel better. After all, a primary function of our life story is to allow us to place difficult experiences firmly in the past and take from them something beneficial that will allow us to thrive in the future. Only when that happens will we know our transition is complete.

—*Bruce Feiler*

There's no better screenwriter of your life story than you, especially in the messiness of midlife. While it may be hard to believe, you understand what brought you to this place in life better than anyone else. You may have been hurt along the way, but, deep down, you know your wounds contain your wisdom. Just find the common thread and show how one action leads to the next. Your story will help me understand my story, since so many of our human themes are common.

Most importantly, the common ingredient in all good storytelling is a love of the story and the characters. And, hopefully, by the time you mature into midlife, you've fallen in love with your story—and the characters in it, including yourself. Or you've at least gained a familiarity with their foibles and missteps that doesn't breed contempt but, instead, compassion.

8.

"I've Learned How to Edit My Life"

*The trip becomes a journey only after
you've lost your baggage.*

Experiencing midlife is a little like being a snake shedding its skin. Just as humans grow out of their clothes, a snake's body grows, but its skin does not. Thus, the snake creates a new, roomier skin layer and molts the old one—along with any harmful parasites that have been clinging to it. As philosopher Friedrich Nietzsche suggests in *The Dawn*, "The snake that cannot shed its skin must perish." As you'll learn in this chapter, this transformation is made infinitely more possible by creating a ritual I call the Great Midlife Edit.

Are you ready for your midlife molt? Shedding our old skin—that veneer we present to the world—isn't easy work. After all, we've often built our life and identity upon a house of business cards. We've made commitments to all kinds of people who are banking on us not to change, not even a little.

Because if we change, they have to change. Of course, challenging times require us to change our habitat—to surround ourselves with other folks who are also ready to experience the rite of passage that gives us the courage to shed our skin.

Disappointment = Expectations Minus Reality

Midlife is the time when we come to terms with the fact that we are never going to be president of the United States, or visit every country on the globe, or win a Grammy. It's when we realize we may not have married our perfect soulmate, our kids aren't going to an Ivy League school, we have far fewer zeros attached to our savings account than we'd expected, or that we'll never get to 25,000 followers on Instagram. But it's also the time when we recognize these aspirations for what they are: fantasies of our younger selves. For me, I've realized I'll never climb Mount Everest, an aspiration I had long ago. And I've made my peace with that.

The collision of youthful expectations with actual reality can be sobering at the start of our midlife years. But it can be a time when we finally free ourselves from the weight of these expectations, let go of our disappointment, and find some peace.

There's social science evidence showing that younger people consistently and markedly overestimate how satisfied they will be in five years, while older people underestimate future satisfaction. Researchers have found that during middle age, our satisfaction with life is declining (that's the U-curve), but our expectations are also starting to decline as well—and that in fact, they tend to decline even faster than satisfaction itself. Eventually, however, expectations settle into a more realistic level than in youth, and reality begins exceeding them. This happens around one's 50s and is part of the reason that life satisfaction begins to rise again.

So, how do you deal with the initial period of disappointments? First, ask yourself, "Am I frustrated or disappointed?" When you are disappointed, it means that all is lost, and the fight has ended. But frustration is the feeling we have when we believe we are still in the game. If you are frustrated (and not disappointed), you can use this energy to alter your reality.

You have two choices when faced with disappointment: improving your reality or lowering your expectations. If you can't alter your reality, the only variable left in this equation is expectation. Many of us find this hard to do. We believe that expectation is what fueled our ambition and success in the first place, so to starve ourselves of that fuel feels like the first step toward learned helplessness. So we thrash away, fueled by frustration, striving to change our reality.

A better way to tame your disappointment is to distinguish between expectation and hope. An expectation is a strong belief that something will happen in the future, while hope is a feeling of optimism, or a wish for that thing to happen. Hope springs eternal, while expectations are often a fleeting fantasy.

Here's another trap to beware of: wrapping an expectation

in entitlement. This is when we mask our disappointment by saying, "Darn, I earned that. Why was it stolen from me?" Whether your business got eviscerated by the pandemic or you've been jilted by your romantic partner, entitlement only ups the ante on your expectations, thus leading to greater disappointment.

So while we welcome greater life expectancy (living longer), we need to be careful with our expectancy about life (longing as a way of living). As the philosopher Seneca writes in *On the Shortness of Life*, "The greatest obstacle to living is expectancy, which hangs upon tomorrow and loses today.... The whole future lies in uncertainty: live immediately."

Letting Go of an Identity Allows You to Create a New One

For so many of us, our midlife expectation reckoning relates to our career. Maybe we haven't advanced as high up the ladder as we once expected, or we're feeling threatened by the new crop of ambitious twenty-somethings who join our ranks every year (we keep getting older, but the new crop is always the same age). Or perhaps work represents the unfortunate combination of maximum productivity with minimum inspiration.

"I am my job." Is there any more American a mantra (spoken or unspoken) than this? I know this worn-out axiom described my own self-concept for most of my adult life. For decades, when someone would ask me how I was doing, I'd immediately talk about how my company is faring. I'll never forget when my friend Vanda cut me off and said, "No, Chipper, I'm asking how YOU are doing."

This can be a difficult question to answer, not just because our career identity sticks to us like an overzealous Band-Aid, but also because by midlife we wear so many roles: parent, child, spouse, colleague, collaborator, citizen. There's a singular YOU and a plural one. So it may be time to consider how many YOUs you inhabit, beyond the YOU in your email signature.

Fortunately, in midlife, we often start to see our professional life (and our ego) from the point of view of a wise observer, hopefully with a dash of humor. We start to recognize that even the words we use to describe our work are toxic. We have "drop-dead" dates. We're "terminated" when we lose our jobs. We're "killing time" at work. When we're doing well, people tell us we're "killing it." Our customers are "target markets." We're "crazy-busy," and our work is considered an "occupation," the same word we use to describe how a foreign country invades its neighbor. We begin to ask ourselves what exactly we were "fighting for" in the first place.

For football legend and MEA faculty member Aaron Taylor, his occupation was his lifeline.

Playing football was a last resort for a teenager who was out of control. He and his single mom, Mardi, moved a lot, so Aaron's childhood was unstable. It was football, and specifically playing for one of America's best-known high school coaches, that brought some structure and self-esteem into young Aaron's life. He went on to attend Notre Dame, where he would later become a College Football Hall of Famer, join the NFL as a first-round draft pick, and win a Super Bowl ring with the Green Bay Packers. What a life, right?!

You can probably guess where this story is going: a series of injuries required him to retire at the ripe old age of 28. He was a VIP, had a fancy car and big house, and was well on his way to financial independence. On paper, he was living the American Dream. But, unfortunately, his whole identity since he was an early teenager had revolved around being a football star.

Professional sports had created the structure and discipline for him to excel. Without the NFL, Aaron's life as a PIP (a Previously Important Person) fell apart—that is, until he got sober and found purpose. He had his midlife transformation way before most of us, but that's often true of those who reach the top of their game in careers that favor the young: pro athletes, fashion models, New York advertising execs, and Silicon Valley software engineers.

Aaron told me,

The first thing I had to do was get honest with myself about what I was going through. I had to own the grief I was experiencing due to the loss of my football identity, as well as the healthy income that fed my fragile ego and elevated my social status. I felt oddly scared, timid, and insecure, because for the first time in my adult life

I wasn't in complete control of my destiny. In the end, it was the lack of purpose, significance, and a vibrant community to call my own that left me feeling like I had lost the most important game in my life... on all fronts.

Aaron's resurrection came when he accepted that he had not only to surrender to his drug and alcohol addiction, but also to let go of his identity as a pro athlete. He discarded his "game face" (as he was having an allergic reaction to that mask) and remade himself into a TV analyst for college football and an advocate for mental health who could share his story with openness, wisdom, and vulnerability. He became a role model once again. But this wouldn't have happened if he'd continued to pine after his past identity as a football star.

You are neither your job, your bank account, nor your shiny car. You are not your trophy wife or husband. You are not even your body. You're something far more wondrous and expansive than that. And midlife is your golden opportunity to shed the masks you have worn for so long.

Ritualizing the "Great Midlife Edit"

Running the midlife marathon is best done without carrying extra baggage. Of course, this is easier said than done.

The first half of life is often about adding and accumulating: not just possessions, or friends, or romantic relationships.

It's also about collecting all those professional roles and titles we've ever held, all the failures, regrets, challenges, and missed opportunities we've experienced, all the stories we've lived and the stories we've told ourselves.

It can be a heavy weight to bear. Try dragging it along with you on this marathon, and you're likely to be worn out by your fiftieth birthday. This is why, as poet David Whyte says, midlife is about "radical simplification."

The compadres who show up at MEA with the greatest sense of need are those who realize it's time for their "Great Midlife Edit." They're sorting through the overstuffed closets of their past, discovering what no longer serves them: what (and who) they can finally shed, whether it's a grudge they've been nursing for decades, the habitual use of alcohol as their primary coping mechanism, a relationship that has outlived its usefulness, or an identity that no longer defines them.

For some, it's coming face-to-face with the fact that they've been living someone else's idea of their life, all while David Byrne's voice rings in their head: "And you may ask yourself, well, how did I get here?" It's remarkable how light and free you feel when you let go of all this baggage.

The first half of life is often defined by the question, "What does the world expect of me?" It's the pursuit of happiness through validation, often with the operating system being one's ego. In contrast, after a week at our Santa Fe Ranch campus, the question I most often hear our alums ask is, "How can I serve the world while also seeking some contentment for myself?" This is a question that speaks to the promise of the second half of life: contentment, curiosity, and service, guided by the operating system of our heart and soul.

MEA alum Connie Michaelis, from Kansas, loves to cook and suggests the editing process we undertake in midlife is like a good reduction method. She says, "Whether you're making a creamy caramel sauce or gravy for the mashed pota-toes, it takes time, heat, a little agitation, all while keeping the lid off, to achieve the perfect flavor. Life is learning to let go of the nonessentials. Just let them burn off and appreciate the rich, sweet reduction that's left." Connie, you've got my taste buds dancing!

Here's a collective ritual we do at the end of the first twenty-four hours of a weeklong MEA workshop, adapted for you to do at home. You're welcome to invite a friend to do this exercise with you, as vulnerability is even more powerful when you share it with someone else.

Start by thinking about where you feel stuck in life, especially if it relates to an expectation you have about yourself. What keeps you up at night? Where do you feel like you've failed? What's a belief you have that's robbing you from living up to your full potential and feeling joy? What's a habit or habitat you're ready to junk? What's a way of being or thinking that used to work, but doesn't anymore?

Take a small piece of paper and write down all the mindsets, habits, and relationships you're ready to let go. Read the list of things you're editing from your life out loud, then light the paper on fire and throw it safely into a bowl or a fireplace. Watch it burn to a crisp (I can't emphasize enough to be safe in doing this exercise. I DO want you to have a second half of your adult life).

Then, take out another piece of paper and list the mindset, habits, or relationships you'll be adding to your life to replace what you've just edited. For example, if you wrote, "I'm terrible at yoga" as a mindset you want to edit, the replacement mindset might be "I love how I feel at the end of a yoga class." Or if you wrote, "I will never be as successful as I used to be in my career," you might replace that with "I will define a new way to measure success in my career." Don't burn this piece of paper. Save it and savor it. It is a guide for your future.

What are you ready to let go of in pursuit of a better (second half of) life?

Knowing What to Notice — and What Not to Notice

We started this chapter with a quote from a wise philosopher, and we'll end with one. William James writes, "The art of being wise is the art of knowing what to overlook." There's a delicious freedom in learning what to edit from our lives. One benefit is that it frees up space to focus on what's been "under-looked."

Often, these are the quiet joys that have crept further and further away from the center of our lives and awareness, shoved aside by the seemingly more urgent demands of our goals, responsibilities, and to-do lists. In Woody Allen's film *Manhattan*, often considered an ode to his hometown, New York City, and a potent depiction of looming midlife crisis (his character, 42-year-old Isaac Davis, is dating 17-year-old

Tracy in the film), there's a scene in which Davis tries to figure out what makes life worth living, and he lists everything from Groucho Marx to Louis Armstrong to "those incredible apples and pears by Cézanne."

Midlife is the time to rediscover our love of old movies, jazz music, impressionist painters, and anything else that makes life worth living. If I were to make a list of what's been under-looked in my life, it might include sunset walks with my dog Jamie in Baja, playing hide-and-seek with my sons in our tropical palm orchard, listening to *The Miseducation of Lauryn Hill*, slow rambles through Balinese rice fields, the Telluride Film Festival, the scene with the swirling plastic bag in the wind in *American Beauty*, reading the Sunday *New York Times* in the bath while listening to any Ennio Morricone soundtrack, my mom's spaghetti.

When we let go of that which is no longer serving us, it's remarkable what can emerge, including an appreciation for all the things we love in our lives. It's sadly remarkable just how much of our adult life is spent trying to solve our problems or toil in ways that don't nourish us. This is the time of your life when you can find the space to stop and smell the roses. Better yet, you can plant some roses as well.

Now that you've done your Great Midlife Edit, what would be on your list of things that make life worth living?

THE
VOCATIONAL
LIFE

9.

"I'm Joyously Stepping off the Treadmill"

Midlife is when we outgrow our pursuit of
happiness and start our practice of joy.

When I hear the word *mantra*, I typically think of a word or phrase that one silently repeats to aid concentration during meditation. In fact, the word is derived from two Sanskrit words: *man*, which refers to the mind, and *tra*, which means "tool" or "means." So the literal definition of *mantra* is "a tool of the mind." Sounds quite liberating, right?

But, then, there are the mantras that we subconsciously repeat to ourselves, often through pure habit, rather than intention: those nagging voices in our heads that we just can't seem to quiet. These mantras, or mindsets, can be anything but a tool to open our minds, especially if they're accompanied by obsessive "pursuit" (which literally means a "chase with hostility"). Instead of liberating, they can confine how we show up in life.

The first half of life is often defined by four mantras/ mindsets:

- "I AM what I do." (achievement)
- "I AM what others say about me." (image)
- "I AM what I have." (status)
- "I AM what I control." (power)

How has the first half of your adult life been defined by these mindsets? How might you rank them in terms of their influence on how you've lived your life?

It's around midlife that many of us realize that these mantras are roadblocks to living a good life. We jump on our metaphorical treadmills, chasing these mantras, and, while they may have served us, they now feel like empty calories. They're not feeding our joy. Instead of the mind, they are tools of the ego, distracting us with the pursuit of recognition and validation from others. But in midlife, we begin to reconsider whether it's more important to be *well known* by the masses OR to be *known well* by those we really care about.

When we perceive time horizons as shorter and more limited, we stop sprinting on the treadmill toward some distant future destination and allow ourselves to stand still and appreciate where we are in the present. We also start to more deeply consider what impact we're having on those closest to us as well as our community more broadly.

What if your new mantra starting at midlife was, as developmental psychologist Erik Erikson suggests, "I am what survives me"? What kind of purpose, legacy, and impact on future generations might sprout out of this alternative perspective?

Try sitting down one weekend when you have a little extra time for reflection. Imagine that you've been handed a ledger to account for your life: who are you, what do you stand for, who have you helped, what seeds have you planted, and how do you want to be remembered? Make a list of what will survive you and how you might invest more in this part of your life moving forward.

Are You Afflicted with "Successism"?

The word *consumerism* is 70 years old and refers to a very American desire to "keep up with the Joneses" through the accumulation of more and more material goods.

While this addiction to material goods is still alive and well in our society, we're also battling a newer and arguably more dangerous addiction: "successism," which refers to the pursuit of ever more success in a manner that is damaging to our well-being and dignity. Midlife is when most of us wake up to the fact that neither consumerism nor successism will bring us happiness and decide that it's time to rewrite our own "success script."

In childhood, almost all of us were issued a success script by our parents and family, our peers and community, and the messages we received from society at large. Some of us deserved an Oscar for how well we inhabited our role in this play. Others rejected the script and rebelled. Whichever camp you fell into, midlife is the time to write a new script that feels more authentic to you. One that isn't written or directed by someone else.

As someone who has been "mainlining success" most of my life, it was revelatory when I was introduced to the shadow side of my success script:

- The sacrifices I made in relationships.
- The stress I felt when trying to measure up to my business school friends.
- The momentary adrenaline high I felt after succeeding at something but that only lasted until something new captured my attention.
- The narcissistic desire to impress.
- The feeling that I was only as valuable as my most recent success.

For those who subscribe to this mindset, success is like a toll road we can take to avoid the congested highway of common life. We pay extra to be on this road, however: through the literal cost of our education, the opportunity cost of sheer number of hours we work, and the stress we experience on the "hedonic treadmill" that allows us to feel like we're a "success," however we define it.

This treadmill is alluring, but it's also deceiving. A

treadmill keeps you running in place, even if you're sprinting. You feel like you're exerting so much effort and maybe you're catching up to your short-term goals, but once you do, it doesn't give you the jolt of joy you were looking for. So you see your next destination on the horizon and off you go again, without stopping to ask what exactly it is that you're sprinting toward.

If this feels familiar to you, I heartily recommend you read Tennessee Williams's *New York Times* essay "The Catastrophe of Success," written in 1947, three years after his first major play, *The Glass Menagerie,* was a huge hit. In it, he describes how his sudden fame and success took away his humanity, leaving cynicism and a distrust of other people in its place. Success fueled his desire for more success until he found himself ordering room service alone in swanky hotel rooms, seriously unhappy. The catastrophe of success likely explains, at least partially, the many pop-culture icons who took their own lives (many of them in midlife) in recent years: Robin Williams, Kate Spade, Anthony Bourdain, Margot Kidder, David Foster Wallace, Amy Winehouse.

It's around midlife that we start to wonder what the heck we're doing on this concrete superhighway, and choose instead to take gorgeous country roads with no toll. We realize that instead of putting our heads down and sprinting to nowhere, we can slow down and enjoy the scenery around us instead.

Author David Brooks suggests that around midlife we experience a motivational shift, which he calls the Second

Mountain. Instead of chasing after the new, shiny object—the fancy job title, the prestigious award—we're more focused on our own character formation as well as on the well-being of those around us. This is how successism loosens its grip on us.

Discovering What Was Meant to Be

Irene Edwards is a successful type-A Filipina American who became the editor in chief of *Sunset* magazine in her early 40s. It's what she'd always dreamed of, ever since she was 13 and got the chance to visit the offices of *Vanity Fair* magazine on a school trip, and decided right then and there that she wanted to be a magazine editor.

And so she leapt right on that treadmill and cranked the speed up to extra high. Summer internships, journalism school, then right after graduation, one job after another at some of the most esteemed publications in the United States. By the time she finally achieved the career goal she'd dreamed about for so long—becoming editor in chief at a major magazine—she had run herself ragged. It didn't help that the industry was barely holding together at the seams.

She was leading a brand and a team that she dearly loved, but was handed a mandate to maximize the bottom line—forcing her to make some difficult and painful choices, including, ultimately, to lead the sale of the magazine, which came with even more turbulence and heartache. When it was all over, she knew her career in media was done—and so was the aspirational identity she had so carefully nurtured and cherished for more than thirty years.

Along the way, she realized she was sacrificing her wellbeing and her relationship with her family, but she didn't see any other choice. As a young person in New York City — and in the cutthroat *Devil Wears Prada* world of magazine publishing, no less — successism had been the norm. And, given how much energy and motivation she'd had back before she got married and had two kids, she hadn't minded running herself ragged in pursuit of excellence.

As is true of so many people who have been running on the treadmill for so many years, by the time Irene approached her mid-40s, she felt as if her life had cracked into pieces. And when she took a long hard look at the damage and disappointment she'd caused herself and others, she did not like what she saw. She knew she was more than this career that she had built and that was now over.

Her first act had come to an end, and her second act had yet to be written. In the absence of a carefully crafted storyline, she had to find purpose and joy in something other than those goals she had so lovingly nurtured. The liminal stage seemed to drag on forever — and her progress wasn't linear. Tears were shed, therapy sessions were booked; she spent a lot of time searching for signs. Signs of what? She had no real idea at the time. All she could do was be open to whatever was coming.

Eventually, a new opportunity came knocking. She was offered a job at a design thinking and innovation consultancy filled with brilliant young minds—in Copenhagen, no less. New Industry. New city, new country, new language. New apartment, new schools. New everything. But it came at a time when her family needed an adventure, so off they went.

But it wasn't easy. "I remember one morning soon after we had moved to Copenhagen," she says. "We were sleeping on mattresses and sleeping bags on the floor of our unfurnished apartment, which was quite a step down from the carefully decorated home we had owned in California. My son cried in his pillow at night because he missed his old school. We had been living out of suitcases. I was lonely and homesick."

Luckily she had her wonderful husband by her side. He had always seen the beauty, or at least the humor, in all the everyday things that to her felt difficult and unfamiliar—and he still did. So they'd bundle up, pack a thermos of hot chocolate and provisions for a winter picnic, and go on long bike rides together as a family, exploring their new city.

When the pandemic hit, they hunkered down and created their own daily quarantine routine: family yoga classes in the kitchen in the mornings, remote work/learning in various corners of the apartment, big cozy stews for dinner. Things became so much simpler, in many ways. They had less stuff, but they had more than they needed—most important of all, their close family unit.

With the newfound time and space in which to reflect, the values of Danish society became top of mind for Irene. Systems thinking as a way of daily life. Acting for the common good, rather than for the benefit of the individual. She explains, "Implicit trust in our leaders to have our best interest at heart. All the things that initially seemed rather foreign to me as an American."

Irene now believes that her life is exactly what was always destined to be. She says,

> I'm proud of myself for having had the courage to take my burning trash heap of a midlife and truly rip it all up, trusting there was something else that would take its place. If I could go back in time a couple of years to that sad shell of myself sitting in bed and looking for signs, I would have loved to be able to give her the tiniest of signs that it was all going to be okay. I can't do that, but maybe I can do the next best thing—which is to tell my story, and hope that someone out there reading it takes it as their own sign for the future.

Same Seed, Different Soil

Getting off the treadmill is not an all-or-nothing proposition. Few of us wake up one morning and decide to stop running. More often, it's an evolution; even in midlife, transformation doesn't happen in the blink of an eye. And it takes social support from family and friends to help you ease into a new life.

Sometimes we need to "repot" ourselves in new soil in order to flourish again. I call this phenomenon "same seed, different soil." Over the course of our career, we've developed many seeds of knowledge and wisdom that we can replant in new environments. And as we get older, we are more adept at sensing the kind of habitat in which our seeds will most likely thrive.

By midlife, we may have a blind spot for all the wisdom we've cultivated in a company, in an industry, in a particular position or role; it becomes almost invisible to us, because it's been germinating inside us for so long. Often, it's only when you repot yourself in a new habitat that you start to see what value you can bring to it.

When I joined Airbnb as in-house mentor to cofounder and CEO Brian Chesky, I hadn't fully thought about what it meant to be reporting to my mentee, who was twenty-one years younger than me. Nor had I fully thought about what it would be like to work in a tech company, the land of Millennials, when my whole career up until that point had been in the relatively analog world of boutique hotels.

Thriving in this new soil meant I would no longer be the maverick CEO, the visionary leader, or the "sage on the stage." I was instead the "guide on the side": a role I was not accustomed to playing. As part of my Great Midlife Edit, I had to right-size my ego, knowing that media articles about Airbnb weren't likely to mention me. My success was defined by Brian's success, and my role was to give him the tools to become a world-class leader, not to be one myself.

Beyond the fact that I needed to change my identity from CEO to "CEO whisperer," I also needed to make sure Airbnb was fertile soil in which to plant my seed. It helped that Brian's growth mindset and insatiable curiosity reminded me of my own, as did the alignment I felt with the budding, mission-driven culture of the company.

But what felt most profound about this chapter of my career was something the founders told me a few months into the job: "We hired you for your knowledge, but what we got was your wisdom." It turned out that some of the leadership and EQ basics that I had taken for granted in myself were not so obvious to Millennial entrepreneurs who'd created a billion-dollar company overnight. I'd gotten off the treadmill myself while becoming a leadership fitness trainer for these young, high-potential entrepreneurs.

In a world that is changing faster than ever before, the ability to master transitions has become an essential twenty-first-century skill. So don't let the prospect of unfamiliar soil scare you from exploring what's next. You might be able to plant your seed in many places by thinking of your work life as a portfolio of activities.

Pursuing a Portfolio Career

In Sweden, they call it a smorgasbord. In Hawaii, it's a pu pu platter. In your career, it's a portfolio life. It works like this: Rather than working exclusively for one organization, you work part-time in various capacities—a trend accelerated by the pandemic as the number of global companies offering phased retirement for full-time midlifers more than doubled between 2020 and 2022. If you believe variety is the spice of life, then this may be how you design your work life after age 50.

Stepping off the treadmill doesn't have to mean retiring. It doesn't mean sitting in your living room, watching daytime TV and doing crossword puzzles, trying to find semiproductive ways to fill the long hours in the day. Nor does it mean retiring the knowledge and skills you've worked so hard to build. It simply means reevaluating whether you want to keep chasing the same goals you single-mindedly pursued in your 20s and 30s, and exploring new ways to repurpose all that you have learned.

There are so many options for how to design your portfolio career once you've unshackled yourself from a single full-time job. You might become a consultant, a coach, or professional mentor, a board member, a student back at school, or some combination of these. For many Boomers, the sunset of their career is when they become an entrepreneur. According to a recent Census Bureau's Annual Business Survey, 30 percent of American business owners are between 55 and 64, and another 20 percent are over 65. Wow, who knew that half of American entrepreneurs are 55+?

Here are a few tips for how you might create a Portfolio Career:

1. **Talk with your boss.** Determine if your current employer is open to an extended semiretirement plan for you. Phasing out of your current job could free up

the time to develop other pieces of your portfolio while also providing a stable income.

2. **Become a consultant.** Consider whether your career expertise might be transferable into a consulting career in your industry (though if you are still a part-time employee, you need to be careful that you're not competing with your current employer). You'd be surprised how many people want to know everything you know, especially if you've been working in the same industry for ten, twenty, or thirty years.

3. **Follow your passion.** Assess your hobbies and interests and ask yourself if you could make money as a photographer, a writer, or a coach. When you have multiple streams of income, you have the luxury of earning just $10,000 or $20,000 annually from one of these activities as a piece of your portfolio puzzle.

4. **Monetize your space.** We often have larger living quarters or second homes as we get older. Maybe it's time to consider earning some extra money by becoming a landlord or Airbnb host so that your extra space earns you extra money.

Paula Pretlow had a very active, fruitful career busting through glass ceilings as an African American woman whose single mother decided that her five children would voluntarily desegregate the Oklahoma City public schools during the stormy civil rights era of the late 1960s.

Armed with intelligence and the learned ability to navigate

different and sometimes difficult environments, and with her fearless mother as a role model, Paula built a career in the finance and investment management world at a time where there were very few women, much less women of color. As a divorced single mother and natural community builder, on top of her demanding job, she had a very full life. Until she began to feel burned out and exhausted.

Feeling the need to change course, take a rest, and figure out how to spend the next phase of her life, she decided at age 55 to step away from the company at which she was a partner. Having given her company nearly a year's notice to help prepare for a smooth transition, she was diagnosed with a very serious and aggressive form of breast cancer—one month before her planned exit date. Suddenly, the need for serious reflection became very urgent.

After bilateral mastectomies and successful treatment in an experimental medical trial, Paula decided not to return to corporate life. Instead, she has created a portfolio life to include the things she is most passionate about: making a difference in the lives of people often overlooked and underappreciated AND utilizing all that she learned from her many years in corporate America.

Today, she serves on multiple public and private corporate boards, including one at a Fortune 500 company, and national philanthropic boards, including one whose mission is expanding opportunities in America's cities and another that focuses on meeting basic human needs in priority communities in the United States and Israel.

Paula says, "I've created a portfolio life that allows the precious time I cherish with my family and fulfills my need to make a difference in the world—by bringing a distinctly different voice and lived experience into corporate and philanthropic boardrooms. I'm alive and I'm having a tremendous amount of fun!"

Science has shown that around age 40 or 50, our sense of taste begins to dull. Perhaps variety is just the spice we need to reinvigorate our atrophying taste buds. A portfolio career may spice up your relationship with your work and enhance your life in ways you never imagined.

What Do You Have to Offer?

Author Arthur C. Brooks (no relation to David) says,

The best synthesizers and explainers of complicated ideas—that is, the best teachers—tend to be in their mid-60s or older, some of them well into their 80s. That older people, with their stores of wisdom, should be the most successful teachers seems almost cosmically right. No matter what our profession, as we age, we can dedicate ourselves to sharing knowledge in some meaningful way.

What are the professions that take advantage of our ripening wisdom? Professor? Mediator? Life coach? Author, tour guide, counselor or therapist, consultant, caregiver, religious or spiritual leader, workshop facilitator? Go ahead and add to this list.

A number of recent studies show that general skills, especially soft skills that revolve around emotional intelligence, are more durable than technical ones. So your greatest gifts may lie in the social skills that you've developed over a few decades in the workplace—the kinds of skills that can be learned and lived, but not taught. As a "modern elder," you have great value in the "invisible productivity" you offer: the ability to not just be productive yourself, but to raise the productivity of your mentees and teams.

Psychiatrist and talk-show host David Viscott writes, "The purpose of life is to discover your gift. The work of life is to develop it. The meaning of life is to give your gift away."

Here's an exercise you can do with a partner. Do it in a quiet place where there are no distractions and maybe after you've taken a walk in nature.

Have your partner ask you the following question, "What mastery or gift can you offer?" Answer whatever immediately arises for you. Don't overthink it. The more open you are to any thought that arises, the more likely you are to experience an epiphany. Your partner will say thank you, ask you to take a deep breath or two, and then ask you the same question again. But you're not allowed to answer the same way twice. Open up that channel—wide—and see what flows. Repeat this question five times and see if this archaeological dig unearths some of the mastery you didn't know you possessed.

As I've suggested before, with age comes alchemy. Maybe

your mastery is the combination of two of your identities or skills. Being a lawyer and scientist is much rarer, and more valuable than being only one of those. Finding two skills that you can alchemize is a way to find your unique gift. You don't need to be the very best at either of these things: being in the top 25 percentile in two different skills is easier than trying to be in the top 1 percent of one. Here's an exercise that our MEA alum Douglas Tsoi devised to help you find your recipe for alchemy.

Take a sheet of paper and tear it into strips. On those strips, write down every skill that you're good at (as a benchmark, think of ones you're better at than 75 percent of people). Be generous with yourself; you're good at a lot of things. And think expansively too; you probably haven't thought to include the skills you're good at but take for granted because they seem natural to you. Now take all those strips and put them in a hat. Draw two out at a time. Is the combination of those two skills interesting to you? Keep doing it until you have a few concrete ideas that are valuable and rare to others.

Beware of the "Winner's Curse"

Too often, we enter midlife feeling like a "success machine" that needs a new battery. We've grown accustomed to being very good at what we do and frightened by the prospect of trying something new because who wants to end the last decade or two of their career on a mediocre note? Also, if I stop working so hard, I'm scared my neglected emotions might catch up to me!

This is one reason why people who do well in life often suffer the most as they age. But Arthur Brooks says we need to beware of this "winner's curse." Trying to hang on forever (especially to success) is an exercise in frustration and futility, and limits our new avenues for joy and personal growth.

The onset of a healthy midlife is marked by when we fall into joyous relief that we don't have to base the second half of our life on someone else's definition of success.

A treadmill or stationary bike is a great trainer. Using one is a healthy practice that gives you the illusion you're going somewhere, which is particularly important to someone who sees themselves as a winner. But, around midlife, you realize that the landscape doesn't change around you. You may have the illusion you're winning the race, but you're surrounded by four walls and sweaty bodies in a gym or, outside the metaphor, expectant bodies in a conference room. It's time to get off the treadmill, go outside and enjoy the sun, and start imagining how you might curate your life if you had a little more spaciousness. That's the topic of our next chapter.

10.

"I'm Starting to Experience Time Affluence"

I have time to become a beginner again.

It's amazing how many obligatory commitments disappear once our children leave the nest, we stop sprinting on the career treadmill, we choose to take a midlife gap year, or we trade in city living for the simple joys of smalltown life. Midlife is our opportunity to move from human doing to human being.

Of course, there are times in midlife when we feel like screaming at the top of our lungs, "I'm as busy as hell and I'm not going to take it anymore!" When we're young, we see busyness as a Calvinist virtue: the sign of a rich, full life. But in midlife, we realize that busyness is a form of poverty; it doesn't cost us just our time, but also our space for curiosity, our depth of connection with each other, and our ability to reflect and contemplate. Yet we inflict time poverty on ourselves, based upon the choices we make. The good news is that time affluence is also within our grasp, and we can begin by slowing down time.

How to Slow Down Time

I came late to the podcast craze. The pandemic gave me the space to walk an average of 20,000 steps a day on the beach, in the desert, among the farmland, and in the mountains near my Baja home. I fell in love with podcasts, and they became my occasional companions on my long strolls.

Yet, as leisurely as this time was, given my impatient nature, I wanted to consume an episode quickly. I was worried about having mental indigestion if I listened at 2x the normal speed, but I read a study that said that the human mind can listen to and comprehend words at a rate of about 210 words per minute, which is twice as fast as those same words can be spoken. I became a speed listener and learned fast, but—at the same time—I didn't feel like I savored the experience. And, when I'm listening to Rich Roll, Krista Tippett, or Ryan Holiday, I do want to savor their words. As two of my favorite philosophers say, "There's more to life than increasing its speed" (attributed to Gandhi) and "If I could turn back time..." (Cher).

Our experience of time changes as we age. After all, a year represents 10 percent of a 10-year-old's life but just 2 percent of a 50-year-old's. Researchers explain that we gauge time by memorable events. The more such events, the slower time seems to pass, but because we often have fewer new things to remember as we age, life seems to accelerate. When the passage of time is no longer measured by "firsts" (first kiss, first day of school, first family vacation), the weeks begin to run together, stitched by recurrent and unmemorable daily tasks.

Introducing novelty into your life will make new memories stand out. This is why the best way to slow the passage of time is to become a beginner again.

When I was entering adolescence, I was deeply touched by Harry Chapin's 1974 song "Cat's in the Cradle." At that age, we tend not to think about time slipping away, but this song offered me a "note to self" that has taken on a particular resonance with age: time is one of the most valuable assets we have, and we often learn that too late in our life. Or as Jim Croce says, "There never seems to be enough time to do the things you want to do once you find them."

Chapin's lyrics are about a man who becomes a father and never has enough time for his son. The boy longs for dad time, but also longs to be like his father when he grows up. Finally, when the son graduates from college, the father yearns for quality time with his boy, but the son is too busy. Dad, now retired, reflects after a call with his son, "And as I hung up the phone, it occurred to me he'd grown up just like me. My boy was just like me."

As we age, we start to realize that what's scarce is what's valuable, and time becomes our most scarce asset as we inhabit midlife. Time is a nonrenewable resource. If you spend a dollar, you can make another one. But, if you waste a day, a year, a decade, you don't get it back. The good news is that midlife is a time when we have developed the agency to choreograph our lives to preserve that valuable resource.

Generativity vs. Stagnation

Generativity versus stagnation is the seventh stage of psycho-social development, according to psychologist Erik Erikson. *Generativity* is defined as "the propensity and willingness to engage in acts that promote the well-being of younger genera-tions as a way of ensuring the long-term survival of the spe-cies." In this stage, which we reach in midlife, adults strive to create things, nurture others, contribute to the community, or make some other positive change.

The newfound time affluence we discover in midlife can inspire generativity, or it can lead to stagnation. My college friend, Diane Flynn, is someone who will never stagnate. A successful business leader before leaving the corporate world for sixteen years to raise three kids, she was ready to return to the paid workforce full-time at age 50 but was diagnosed with breast cancer.

Spending months on the couch gave her plenty of time for self-reflection. She carefully considered what filled her tank and what drained her—an exercise she continually practices. She developed a life mantra that has served her well over the past ten years: "I seek to engage in creative collaboration, with people I respect, to change lives and build community." Every opportunity that comes her way passes through the filter of this mantra. She says, "Knowing what you WANT to do, rather than simply what you CAN do is tremendously empowering to find purpose."

Once two of her three kids were off to college, Diane had more time on her hands. She had spent the better half of two decades volunteering at school, the local children's hospital, and serving on nonprofit boards, all of which helped her reenter the workforce and become a role model for other empty-nest moms who had immense talents and lots of time, but a lack of confidence about recharting a professional career.

She launched ReBoot Accel, a program to help midlife women develop the growth mindset necessary to reenter the workforce after having children. And, in the process, Diane came to learn she loved being a speaker, teacher, coach, and facilitator—something she never would have discovered without the benefit of her newfound time.

Diane says,

> I think the world has life backwards. We work like dogs when our kids are young, running around frazzled and having no energy left for relaxation and joy. And then we're expected to retire when we face the empty nest. For me, life after 50 (and after kids have left the house) has been one of the most freeing, energizing times of my life. I have seemingly unlimited time to think, work, play, and enjoy what I'm doing. I just wish as a society that we could all stay home with our families, and then return to work when we have greater wisdom and time.

I've long been a fanboy of Dr. Atul Gawande. This prominent surgeon, Harvard professor, humanist, and health care expert wrote the *New York Times* bestseller *Being Mortal* and was the commencement speaker to Stanford graduate students, where he quoted Dr. Bob Wachter advising a young person, "Say yes to everything before you're 40...and say no to everything after you're 40."

I understand this logic: be open to trying new things when you're young, as you have no idea what's truly going to be important or energizing to you. There's truth to that, but I also believe we're meant to become beginners over and over again in midlife and beyond.

Since Shonda Rhimes wrote *Year of Yes* a few years ago, the world has been possessed by the idea of opting into everything. I love the curiosity and openness in this, but I also wonder about the role of discernment in this thinking. There is something to be said for saying yes more when we're younger and taste-testing the world. When we say yes after 40, we need to add an exclamation point — YES! — because we realize our time is finite.

What are you saying YES! to after 40 years old?

Learning to Become a Beginner Again

Beware of inviting me to a cocktail party! I tend to ask inappropriate questions such as "In what ways are you a beginner right now?" That's quite an opening line, and a beautiful window into how we might improve life by constantly learning, in midlife and beyond. But at a party I often get a quizzical look as folks head for the bar.

Author Tom Vanderbilt, who wrote the book *Beginners*, says as we get older we have the opportunity to move from "knowing that" (the facts of life) to "knowing how" (the experience of life). Too many of us give up the "how" for the "that" because learning *how* to do something new may be more frightening as we age. No one signs up to look like an idiot.

One of our greatest lessons at MEA has been the social value of "being bad" as a beginner among other adult newbies. After all, when you're a beginner in a group of other beginners, being "bad" simply makes you average, allowing you to have fun and develop some skills.

My cofounder Christine Sperber, who is also our Chief Experience Officer, calls this "Type II fun," the kind of activity that, when you're first doing it, can feel a little daunting but that brings you a joyous sense of accomplishment after you've finished. This is why Christine weaves into a workshop week all kinds of activities that might strike fear into one of our workshop participants when they first hear about it: from competitive bread baking to collective improv to the fine art of rock balancing to equine-assisted learning to surfing and yoga (not at the same time).

Babies are not self-conscious when they learn to walk. Yet, as we age, our self-judgment and our ego-preservation rob us of all kinds of opportunities to be a neophyte. It's not easy to learn something new, especially in midlife. Of course, one reason to pursue lifelong learning is to keep our synapses firing in our noggins, but the real value is the pleasure that comes from trying something new.

The goal of becoming a beginner in midlife is not just to get smarter or more proficient at something: it's to approach life with fresh eyes. Becoming a beginner allows us to reengage with and rediscover natural talents we can build at any age. Taking this leap gives us confidence at the exact time we need it most. It turns back the clock. We're perfectly ripe again.

In spite of outward trappings of success, Chris Murchison grew up with an inner voice that never quite believed he was good enough. Growing up as a gay black boy in a homophobic and homogeneous military environment, Chris harbored a secret of scarcity of self. He overcompensated and battled with perfectionism for many years, until he realized, in midlife, that it wasn't working for him anymore.

So he started intentionally immersing himself in new beginnings. This became a transformative growth practice for him—a six-week sabbatical after the grueling experience of implementing an organizational layoff; leaving his job of eleven years to discover his inner artist; taking up bread-making, taiko drumming, and more recently, the art of collage after relocating across the globe from San Francisco to London. He loved becoming a beginner again.

Chris glows when he talks about being a beginner. "Travel, bread, taiko, collage. What they all share is flow. When engaged in each, I have an unusual experience of time—I feel completely engrossed, time slows down and becomes expansive, I get lost in the details and enamored with new-found beauty. It's amazing." He acknowledges that there are challenges, fears, and failures, but says that the process of learning—of stretching himself—increases his confidence. Finally, he has discovered how to accept himself as good enough.

When we are in a state of flow, we lose track of time. And maybe because we lose track of time during those special, ephemeral moments, it is as though our psychological and physical clock stands still. This is just one of the ways becoming a beginner keeps us from feeling stale.

Toward the end of the film *American Beauty*, Kevin Spacey's character drops this exquisite line that speaks to the value of becoming a beginner in midlife, "It is a great thing when you still have the ability to surprise yourself." The line is a profound call to action—urging us to wake up and see the wonder and beauty around us and, more importantly, within us.

What hobbies, skills, or topics have you started exploring for the first time in the past year? What if for the rest of your life you made a commitment to yourself that you would always be a beginner at something?

Recreation or Re-creation?

While recreation and *re-creation* are not mutually exclusive, the latter is the true elixir of life. An alchemical cocktail of curiosity and wisdom, garnished with fresh sprigs of a beginner's mind, creativity, and service. To retire is to withdraw into seclusion. But to re-create is to regenerate, to become new again. In midlife, we start wondering about how we'll spend our golden years. Fewer and fewer of us will be choosing the retirement community with the house on the fairway.

Suzanne Watkins knew she wasn't going to live on a golf course. For years, Suzanne was stuck in her cubicle doing work she didn't love and being a single parent to two kids. She knew she wanted to re-create herself, but she didn't have the time, energy, or perceived freedom. Becoming an empty nester in her 50s finally gave her time to pause, take a step back, and look at her relentless schedule of working three low-paying jobs just to make ends meet. She wanted to see the world but didn't have the savings to do so. Then she had a novel idea of becoming an international flight attendant: she'd be earning an income, learning about an entirely new industry, and best of all, traveling the world for free. So she downsized her lifestyle and passed her flight attendant training around her 60th birthday. She knows that welcoming this transition in her life offered an example to her adult kids that we can re-create ourselves at any age.

Most of us want to leave a legacy, even in the smallest ways. It doesn't have to be your name on a building. It could purely be how you influenced a mentee, cared for your beloved dog, or tended to a community garden in a park near your home. For Suzanne, it's being a role model for her kids. The question we must ask ourselves in middle age is this: will our legacy be one of generativity, or of stagnation?

Here are five questions that could help you define your legacy.

1. Who will be the primary beneficiaries of what I'm leaving behind?
2. What less obvious but more valuable gifts am I leaving?
3. How am I thinking, preparing, and offering this legacy?
4. When would it be most poignant or powerful to ritualize my offer to those who will be here after me?
5. Why am I doing this, and why is it meaningful to me? If it's for my reputation, I've got the wrong idea.

If you can see your own life reflected both in previous and future ones, you know that you are a part of a larger story. There are beautiful films on this subject of legacy from *Schindler's List* to *My Life Without Me* to *It's a Wonderful Life* to *Coco*.

As we curate the gift of time, one of the most important questions we can ask ourselves is, "How can I serve?" It's a question that takes on even greater meaning in midlife and beyond. As a for-profit entrepreneur, I spent the first half of my career focused on Return on Investment (ROI). Now, I'm spending the second half focused on a different form of ROI: Ripples of Impact.

When you drop a pebble in a pond, it creates a series of ripples that cascade out over the water. In our relationships, our emotions can create positive or negative ripples. In our businesses, the choices we make—how we build our company culture, how we affect our community, and how we lead—send energy into the world that will create positive or negative ripples. The same thing is true for how we spend our time. The choice is ours.

With more time in your life, what is your ripple, and how will you share it with the world?

THE SPIRITUAL
LIFE

11.

"I've Discovered My Soul"

Life is a horizontal journey, then a vertical one.

Midday and midlife have a lot in common. Early in the morning, a shadow is cast west. A child dreams about her future. Late in the day, a shadow is cast east. An elder leaves a legacy for future generations. But at midday, with the sun directly overhead, we lose our shadow, just as we may lose our sense of direction in midlife. This is a temporary condition, as the afternoon will eventually reemerge, but our midlife circumstances and emotions aren't as predictable as the sun.

You may be feeling the impact of a midday midlife. You may feel a little lost or stuck, like you're missing your compass. You may feel like you're supporting everyone else and tending to their needs so much that you've lost track of your own. You may be bored silly. You may feel questions about the meaning of life slipping through the cracks of your over-packed calendar. You may be seeking solitude more than you did five years ago. You may find yourself becoming an introvert.

All of this can be disorienting. But don't fret. A new primary operating system is being installed in your life, upgrading you from the era of the ego to the stage of the soul. What may feel like a rupture may lead to a rapture. This is why, in midlife, many of us turn inward: we realize that our soul needs space, solitude, and quiet. Or perhaps it's that *we* need space, solitude, and quiet to reconnect with our soul.

Where is your monastery of consciousness, the place where your soul gets to breathe?

As we age, it is natural to intuitively retreat from the social world. Maybe that was a silver lining of the pandemic when "social distancing" forced a little "soulful listening." This is a time to stop looking for answers and instead to notice what questions are stirring so you become present to the pull of your soul.

I know this may be an unfamiliar language to you. Maybe it's meant to be an inner nudge or a pull to your heart. If you've gotten this far along in the book, you know that midlife is bereft of a common language. While the awakening of early adulthood was loud, unmistakable, and full of social rituals that helped to solidify our external identity, the awakening of mid-adulthood is subtle, internal, and socially invisible.

In his book, *Falling Upward: A Spirituality for the Two Halves of Life*, Richard Rohr writes,

> There is much evidence on several levels that there are two major tasks to human life. The first task is to build a strong "container" or identity; the second is to find the contents that the container was meant to hold.... The language of the first half of life and the language of the second half are almost two different vocabularies, known only to those who have been in both of them.

One piece of language I introduced earlier in the book was "middlescence," this era when we're going through the adult counterpart to adolescence. Maybe middlescence is the time when our internal operating system shifts from the ego to the soul, yet we are given no manual for navigating this shift. Well, that's why I wrote this midlife manifesto. To help guide you on this journey to your soul.

The Bookends of the Ego

It is sometimes said that the first half of life is devoted to forming a healthy ego, while the second half is going inward and letting go of it.

In childhood, our souls are filled with wonder, often at one with the people and the natural world around us. And, then, as we transition into adolescence, a psychological phenomenon occurs. The ego, which emerged early in life as a means of staking our place in the world, becomes a driving force. We drive that powerful operating system straight into adulthood, some of us revving our engines and others trading in our vehicle for a sportier, younger model. No doubt, our ego is on full display in our 20s, 30s, and 40s.

Is it possible that what we've labeled "midlife crisis" since 1965 is just a profound change in our operating system for the rest of our lives? Could it be that adolescence and middlescence represent the bookends of the ego?

People often refer to midlife and beyond as the "golden years," but they are also the "emboldened years," the years when we're emboldened to shove the ego out of the way and allow the soul to take over.

It's almost like we're being asked, in the middle of our lives, to trade in our car with an automatic transmission for one with a stick shift. At the same time, we're also being asked to drive that stick-shift car on the steep hills of San Francisco in the rain, while trying not to stall. Not easy!

Fortunately, as we start to build some familiarity with our new way of driving, we come to realize that driving a stick is a tactile and engaging experience. It feels like there is more connection between the driver and the machine, between our soul and our physical being. Suddenly, getting to where we want to go becomes more liberating and infinitely more enjoyable.

Welcome to your midlife driving school. Let's test-drive your soul.

Stand Up and Show Your Soul

This may sound daunting, but just as you first learned to drive in a parking lot or on a country road, the sprouting of your soul can happen in small, manageable, yet meaningful ways.

Author Clarissa Pinkola Estés captures this perfectly. She suggests that our role is not to fix the world, but to focus on what we can do that is within our grasp. And doing that spurs on other people. She writes, "One of the most calming and powerful actions you can do to intervene in a stormy world is to stand up and show your soul." Such powerful words, especially in these disorienting times. The infectiousness of a shining soul cannot be overestimated, especially in dark times. Your courage gives me courage, and mine ignites courage in someone else who catches a glimpse of my soul. It is this movement of our soul that creates a global movement and fuels the necessary catalyst for us to rise up in unison. Each of us is a role model, even if we think no one is watching.

The soul needs meaning as nourishment. Meaning can come in many forms, but it often comes in the form of service. Through service, you discover a greater sense of who you are and what you're capable of—because you're being guided by your soul instead of your ego.

In early midlife, I joined the board of the Glide Memorial Church, a Methodist congregation located in San Francisco's Tenderloin district, led by Reverend Cecil Williams, an African American liberation theology activist who gained a global reputation for tending to the poor. I joined the church in my late 20s because my first hotel was located just a few blocks from Glide.

I loved that the Sunday celebrations were radically inclusive, full of people from all walks of life. The rollicking gospel music that emanated from its walls turned Glide into a tourist attraction—especially since it was across the street from the biggest hotel in San Francisco. And Cecil's sermons were legendary.

I'd been on many nonprofit boards before and have to admit that I was occasionally that well-meaning jerk who wanted to prove he was the smartest guy in the boardroom, partly because I was the youngest. My ego was on full display.

But there was something about the Glide board that was different. I was, once again, the youngest one in the boardroom, but I also noticed the character of my elders. Not one was there for their ego. All of us volunteered to regularly serve lunch to the community that lined up on the streets for hours. I loved how I left board meetings feeling enlivened and awake, rather than obsessed with how I'd performed.

Over time, Cecil started asking me to come onstage with him on Sundays to "lift the offering," a means of encouraging congregants to contribute as the baskets for donations were passed around. Of course, this was a little scary, speaking to an audience of 1,000 people. But my stage fright melted away when Cecil and his wife, Jan, reminded me, "This is not about you, Chip. It's your story that will serve Glide." Once I got the hang of it, I found it cathartic, especially when I was going through my darkest times. I think Cecil knew that so he asked me to lift the offering a couple of times each year.

Near the end of my tenure on the board, in my early 50s, one of the co-pastors sent me an email saying Cecil wanted me to tell my story that Sunday. Of course, I thought this meant lifting the offering again. I said yes and didn't think much of it until that morning, when I showed up at the church ten minutes before the first of two services was to begin and ran into Cecil, who said, "How does it feel to be giving today's sermon, Chip?" Wait a minute—I didn't realize that's what I was being asked to do!!

When you give Glide's sermon, not only do you have to speak for twenty minutes—twice—you sit onstage next to Cecil for both services, which meant that I had no time to go hide in a bathroom stall and write my first sermon. I told Cecil that I had no idea what I was going to say up there, and he just repeated what he'd told me many years ago: "This is not about you, Chip. It's your story that will serve Glide." And then he added, "Have fun out there."

During the next thirty minutes, as I sat onstage next to Cecil, feeling not at all ready for sermon time, I stared at the stained-glass windows and remembered a saying: "We're all broken. That's how the light gets in." I felt this wrestling match between my ego, which wanted to get it right, and my soul, which wanted the light to shine in.

By the time I stepped to the pulpit with no notes and nothing memorized, I could feel that, with the help of a little "Miracle-Gro" from Cecil, my soul had outgrown my ego. I offered the congregation my personal story, not as the "sage on the stage," but as the flawed and evolving human that I am.

Author Jett Psaris writes, "Rather than an opponent of the soul on the battlefield of life, the ego has been a reflection all along of the more spontaneous, authentic possibility of who we can be when we are soul-centered; in fact, the ego is the soul in a primitive, undeveloped state."

The ego and the soul, she says,

> share the same existence just as coal and diamonds are both pure carbon. But coal must go through a tremendous transformation, during which time it is subjected to high temperatures and incredible pressure, before its atomic structure is reordered into the pattern of the crystal that we know as a diamond.

She goes on to liken this process to how the tremendous stress placed on the ego, facilitated by midlife experiences, transforms it into something new and brilliant: the soul.... And so that midlife shift in our operating system "depends on our ability to allow the soul to evolve beyond the ego structure encasing it."

That's enlightening, isn't it? The ego and the soul are not at war. And once we "liberate ourselves from the conditioned rigidity, predictability, and density of our ego identities," as Jett writes, "we shift toward being lighter, more transparent, and conscious, as we come to realize that our souls are the true, essential part of us, lying beneath who we have believed ourselves to be."

The Accidental Soul Man

Jeff Hamaoui and his wife, Rachel, had been living in Northern California for twenty years. They had two young children and all the trappings of a meaningful life. The two of them ran their own consultancy focused on sustainability, community development, and systems change: a company with a mission, as well as a global footprint and some amazing clients. They had purpose in their work, people in their lives that they loved and admired.

Yet, as Jeff surveyed his life in his mid- to late 40s, something wasn't quite right. He had the sense that he and his family were, in the words of U2, "running to stand still," and in need of a "systems upgrade." He and Rachel had everything they could have hoped for from the traditional American Dream, but the pressure of keeping it was relentless. Cracks were showing in their relationship, their mental health, and, to top it off, the children they had worked so hard to bring into their lives were being raised by a nanny. As Jeff put it, "Our lives made no sense."

Clearly, it was time for a change. It took them a year to make a big shift, leaving the Bay Area and taking an open-ended sabbatical from their work. They chose to drive south because Baja enticed Jeff with the promise of plentiful surfing.

Surfers often talk about the sport as being spiritual. In fact, entire books have been written on the subject. For Jeff, being in nature, being in flow, watching large animals glide through the ocean and the large raptors patrol the skies along the shore, experiencing the epic twinkling of "god light" that lances through the cloud and fog in a typical Northern California morning all combined into what felt like a spiritual experience. And he loved the "congregation," the community of surfers who were similarly devoted to this craft of catching a majestic wave.

Jeff had studied religious philosophy at university and was drawn more broadly to the spiritual world, but his experience of spirituality through a largely Western lens was mediated by individuals and institutions he didn't trust. His early experiences with both the Jewish and Anglican faiths boggled his mind with their never-ending rules and rituals. As a free thinker, he found the rigidity and contradiction of such belief systems completely incompatible with the workings of his mind.

Arriving in Baja, Jeff was instantly forced to confront spirituality from a very different perspective. Far from being institutionalized, the spirituality in Baja is ingrained in the experience of the place itself. The ocean, the mountains, the endless skies, the dazzling stars, and the superabundance of nature inspire a kind of daily reverence that you almost have no choice but to participate in. Surfing became the closest thing he had in his life to a spiritual practice, and he was religious in his adherence to his weekly surf rituals and rites.

This "wild spirituality" is a daily part of life in Baja. Mexican culture is riddled with magic, shamanism, and an everyday lived spirituality that was incredibly foreign to Jeff. Foreigners attracted to Baja are often explorers, open to cobbling together their own belief systems and practices into their own configurations and on their own terms. Gods and gurus had little to offer Jeff well into his 40s, but Baja was the perfect incubator in which to explore and imagine his own spirituality again.

When Jeff arrived at the MEA to take part in its very first beta workshop cohort, he was intimidated by the meditation, yoga, and mindfulness of it all but appreciated that the community and cofounders (Christine Sperber and I) weren't dogmatic about MEA's spiritual principles and practices.

Jeff started facilitating some of the beta workshops and proved to be world-class in his ability to channel wisdom as something that isn't taught, but is shared. And he started to see that mindfulness practices could include surfing, gardening, and cooking dinner with friends. He started to see that many of his pastimes and passions — not just surfing — could become his religion, and that the mundane could be sacred. Soon, Jeff became the third cofounder of MEA.

In that first year, Jeff built a close relationship with an MEA neighbor and faculty member, Dr. Dacher Keltner, the author of *Awe: The New Science of Everyday Wonder and How It Can Transform Your Life*. In research that drew on thousands of interviews across twenty-six countries, Keltner and his team had identified eight major pathways to awe. Ranked according to which path generates the most awe across cultures, they are:

1. Moral beauty (kindness, courage, etc.)
2. Collective effervescence
3. Nature
4. Music
5. Visual design
6. Spirituality
7. Contemplating life and death
8. Epiphanies (important realizations)

These findings were truly surprising to Jeff, as they suggested there were so many paths to the divine. He says, "I have spent most of my adulthood with a resistance to the idea of divinity. Recently, in a moment of clarity, I realized that faith, for me, in among the profusion of life and beauty, is not really in question. If I want to have faith that there is something greater than myself all I need to do is open my eyes and see the world as it really is."

He continues,

I realized my struggle was with grace. From my own exploration, grace is the understanding that you have a natural place in the scheme of divinity. As I evolve my own thoughts and feelings on this, I believe that anything that brings us into communion with life and the natural world, with other people and the grace with which we can move in the world, is an opportunity to be in relationship, to understand ourselves as part of that divinity and to feel one's soul.

And, so, my good friend Jeff found his soul, even though he wasn't looking for it. His story is not that unusual for those in midlife. Maybe our soul finds us at this age.

Who Is Your Midwife for Midlife?

I think you have to grow up twice. The first time happens automatically. Everyone passes from childhood to adulthood, and this transition is marked as much by the moment when the weight of the world overshadows the wonder of the world as it is by the passage of years. Usually you don't get to choose when it happens.

But if this triumph of weight over wonder marks the first passage into adulthood, the second is a rediscovery of wonder despite sickness, evil, fear, sadness, suffering—despite everything. And this second passage doesn't happen on its own. It's a choice, not an inevitability. It's something you have to deliberately go out to find, value, and protect.

—Magician Nate Staniforth

In midlife, our tastes are changing. Our balance has shifted. Our voice is becoming resonant. I like to think of it as not just second nature, but "second nurture," a time when we nurture our souls by connecting with something deeper.

Midlife is the time for an intentional spiritual rebirth.

I've always thought being a midwife—helping birthing mothers bring a precious, new life into the world—must be a glorious, strenuous calling. Midlife is almost like our second birth, but where are the midwives to help guide us through our midlife labor?

Richard Rohr suggests that our midlife midwives are all around us. He writes, "The midwife of the spirit is not an expert called in for the dramatic moments.... Like a midwife, she works with the whole person and is present throughout the whole process.... She offers support through every stage and waits with the birth-giver when 'nothing is happening.'"

I understand this way too well, based upon the darkest time of my life. I was starting a drive to the Golden Gate Bridge to ponder a jump in 2009 when two midwife angels appeared in my life. As I drove, I called my friend Vanda, who was well aware of how my life was falling apart, and told her how destroyed and defeated I felt that fateful evening. Fortunately, she was trained as a muse and wisdom worker, so she was well prepared for midwifery. Vanda's years spent with people at the end of their lives is what informs her ability to midwife midlife transitions. It just helped to know she was there for me during my time of need.

I parked the car, bawling my eyes out, listening to my

midwife. As Vanda was reminding me why life was worth living, Aretha Franklin's "Amazing Grace" magically showed up on my SiriusXM radio dial. I felt as though Clarence, the angel who saves Jimmy Stewart from jumping off a bridge in *It's a Wonderful Life*, was alive and well.

I'm glad to still be living to tell you that the butterfly can emerge from the darkest chrysalis.

Who is there for you as you shift your operating system from your ego to your soul? How might you be a midwife for midlife for someone else?

12.

"I Feel as If I'm Growing Whole"

*I'm here to be me, which is taking a great deal
longer than I had hoped.*

—*Anne Lamott*

In the first half of our lives, our "selves" are compartmentalized: the person we are at work is often different from the person we are with our spouses and kids. We have certain fragments of ourselves that we show to our oldest friends, and entirely different fragments we show to acquaintances we have just met. In midlife, however, the whole becomes bigger than the sum of its parts as we start to learn to integrate all of who we are.

Many wise philosophers have suggested that our aging process is meant to reveal the beauty that has always been hidden inside us. Perhaps, if we recognize (and accept) that our inner beauty shines brighter as we age, fewer of us would worry about being old. We would come to realize that our purpose in midlife is to emulate the sculptor Michelangelo, who unlocked David from the stone.

Yes, we are in the process of growing old, but we're also growing whole. And we aren't just whole individually, but we're part of a larger whole. Freed from the harness of social pressure and expectations, we start catching a glimpse of the unexpected pleasures of aging and feeling part of something bigger.

Maybe aging is our curriculum for becoming more conscious. And, in our process of becoming more conscious, we become more present, more integrated with ourselves and everyone and everything around us. It's like we've been wearing blinders much of our life. The process of learning to become whole is taking off those blinders.

Growing and Aging Are the Same Thing

We're comfortable saying to a 15-year-old, "My, how you've grown!" but we'd never say that to a 65-year-old. And, of course, we will never say to that 15-year-old, "Wow, you've aged since I last saw you."

When does growing stop and aging begin? Is it 25, 45, 65? That's a loaded question because it suggests you can't grow and age simultaneously.

Having lived in the San Francisco Bay Area for nearly forty years, I know the majesty of a towering redwood, the tallest tree on the planet. They can span more than 400 feet, which is taller than a thirty-seven-story skyscraper. A typical redwood lives for 500 to 700 years, although some coastal redwoods reach the age of 2,000 years, according to the National Parks Service. Not only that, but coastal redwoods have been on the planet far longer than humans. They've been around for over 240 million years, which means they inhabited the earth at the same time as the dinosaurs.

We have wrinkles. Trees have rings. These growth rings not only tell us its age, they offer clues about the climate conditions the tree lived through. Our wrinkles are the same. The only difference is that we don't grow taller as we acquire more wrinkles, whereas trees continue to both age and grow.

In a forest, nutrients tend to flow from the oldest to the youngest trees. A small seedling tree that has been severed from the forest's underground circuitry is much more likely to die than one that is part of a rooted network. And, as a tree nears its death, it bestows its carbon on its neighbors. This is a good metaphor for the knowledge and wisdom that we can bestow on the younger generation as we age.

When it comes to nature, we marvel at the grace and majesty of the old. We see the trees that stretch to the heavens, enraptured with their beauty and "old growth."

What if we applied that same thinking to older humans? What if we looked at them (and ourselves) and saw the grace and beauty that comes with age? And what if we saw their wrinkles as testimony to their internal growth—the growth of heart, spirit, and soul—like we do the rings of a tree? How many rings do you have inside you?

Tragically, when we apply the term *old growth* to humans, it sounds like an oxymoron. Old people don't grow; they just die. Yet every living thing dies at some point, and most animals and trees wear their years much as we do.

Growing and aging are not mutually exclusive, neither in redwoods nor in humans. In the forest, growth requires regeneration—of old leaves, of old branches, of anything that needs composting. In humans, it requires the regeneration of old ideas, old identities, of any part of our life that needs reimagining. It is that cycle of life and death that makes an ecosystem so fresh and alive.

So, if we could realize that our earthly body isn't the only way to measure growth, we'd realize that our hearts and souls continue to learn and grow all the way up to our last breath. And that's when we would realize that *old* and *growth* can be synonymous.

What if you were to make a list of all the ways you're still growing today? Once you've finished that list, make a list of all the ways you hope you're still growing near the end of your life.

Wholeness Is a Path to Holiness

Wholeness is a feeling of being connected with something bigger than ourselves. And growing old is about growing whole and, sometimes, holy.

We are in harmony with nature when we're whole. When we're integrated, not fused. Richard Rohr says,

How do you know if you are on a path that leads to increasing wholeness and involves living out of wholeness? You will hear harmony, not simply the cacophony of a fragmented self. You will also sense the energy of the larger whole—an energy that goes beyond your own. You will, at least occasionally, experience the thrill of being simply a small part of a large cause.... We live wholeness when we "re-member" our story and, through it, experience a deeper sense of being part of a greater whole.

As we age, we reassemble ourselves. We identify the "breadcrumbs" in our lives and how they've led us down a path to wholeness and holiness: a path that has allowed us to bear witness to something much bigger and more profound than ourselves.

I've long had an admiration for the physician and scientist Dr. Phil Pizzo. As a son of immigrant parents and the first in his family to attend college, his career has focused on caring for others, whether by advancing life-saving research on childhood cancers and AIDS, serving as the Dean of Stanford Medical School, or creating the Stanford Distinguished Careers Institute (DCI) that I mentioned in the first chapter.

He's also completed multiple marathons, runs ten miles a day, and finishes a book every week due to the fact that he listens to audiobooks while he runs. He's a rebellious thinker with a mild-mannered, self-effacing way of moving through the many different worlds he inhabits. It was in his late stage of midlife that he felt the calling to integrate those worlds.

At age 77, he surprised quite a few of us when he announced he was studying to become a rabbi, especially since he was raised Roman Catholic and had converted to Judaism only a couple years earlier. As is true with so many people later in life, he could see the through line of his journey—life-long caring, learning, healing, and inquiring—as movements in a splendid symphony, building momentum toward his crescendo.

He's curious about the connection between physical and spiritual healing, between science and religion, and between pastoral counseling and his own contemplative practice. While some might see his next chapter as a life-changing departure from his past, he sees it as an integral part of his story, especially given that he believes he still has so much life still ahead of him.

Fifty-year-old Doug Lynam has been on the path toward wholeness—and holiness—his entire life. In early adulthood, he traded in his life as a hard-core Marine to become a Benedictine monk. However, by midlife, he felt suffocated and even traumatized by monastic restrictions, which he felt hindered further spiritual growth. He found the rules and structure of a religious community helpful for the first half of his life, but they became a barrier to embracing the wisdom and radical freedom of elderhood in the second half.

In his quest for greater meaning and integration, Doug took a leap of midlife faith and left the monastery after twenty years of service to become a money manager focusing on environmentally and socially responsible investing. In addition to his work helping build a more just, sustainable, and participatory economy, he channeled his contemplative wisdom into compassionate action by founding an entheogenic church—a nondenominational, interfaith house of worship that incorporates the safe use of plant medicine into its religious practice. He now helps clients, friends, and parishioners heal themselves through plant-based medicine journeys, and is at one with himself, which may be the ultimate luxury in life.

Finding Presence Under a Tree

Unfortunately, most of us don't break out of our comfort zones before we are forced to do so. Poet David Whyte suggests we are living four or five years behind the curve of our own transformational frontier.

He continues,

> People usually only come to this frontier when they have had a terrible loss in their life or they've been fired or some other trauma breaks open their story. Then they can't tell that story any more. But having spent so much time away from what is real, they hit present reality with such impact that they break apart on contact with the true circumstance.

But what if we could approach this frontier without having external circumstances force us out of our comfort zones?

One thing I've learned from the indigenous people I've met in Mexico and New Mexico is that they are often far less fixated on the past or future than they are on the present. They're fascinated with what's in front of their noses—whether it's a technicolor sky or the emotional state of a family member. They are not four or five years behind—they are in the present moment.

Long ago, when I asked my favorite shaman, Saul, for advice on becoming more present, he said, "Find presence under a tree." And this from a Jewish shaman! I teased back, "I didn't know you celebrated Christmas—?" Saul smiled at my cheekiness, but he knew I knew what he meant: that quiet and calm were waiting for me in the solace and beauty of nature. I just had to make time for it. I had to sit with it. I had to let go and pay attention to what matters.

I have taken Saul's words to heart, especially when I resist them the most. When I feel that compulsive urge to go faster, do more, and be more, it is my cue to immediately put a little "spying on the divine" time in my calendar. I sit under a tree until I am breathing slower and walking slower and until I am where I need to be—fully present within myself. I know that only then will I be fully present for my family, friends, loved ones, and all who come into my life.

The opposite of presence is absence. It's a modern condition, caused largely by our preoccupation with our devices. It's also a condition caused by dementia and Alzheimer's, those afflictions we so fear later in life. We all want to live healthier and longer. But what's the point of a long, healthy life if we're not truly present for it?

How are you welcoming more presence in your life? How could you spend thirty minutes less online per day and use that time to find presence in nature, through meditation, by journaling?

Pressing "Play" on Your Life Again

It has been said you can discover more about a person in an hour of play than in a year of conversation. So true. I can't tell you how many MEA alumni have told me that they experienced more transformation in a week's workshop than they did in years of therapy. There is deep value in letting our mirror neurons play and dance together so we can feel that wholeness of who we are in the presence of others.

Sociologist Émile Durkheim coined the term "collective effervescence" to describe the magic of those moments when our sense of ego separation dissolves and is replaced by communal joy. He writes, "The very act of assembling is an exceptionally powerful stimulant. Once the individuals are assembled, their proximity generates a kind of electricity that quickly transports them to an extraordinary degree of exaltation."

In the wake of five friends committing suicide in midlife, followed by my own dark night of the soul, I became curious about collective effervescence. I'd experienced that kind of wholeness as a founding member of the Burning Man board of directors. Out on what we call the "playa" in the Nevada desert, I saw how a community can support the holistic health of its members through rituals and revelry. At age 50, during a time when I was going through deep uncertainty, I made a list of experiences I'd had in the past couple years that enlivened me, and found that many of them involved experiencing communal joy.

So, just after I sold my hotel company and before being asked to join Airbnb, I decided to take a gap year (my midlife atrium) dedicated to exploring communal joy, and over that year I attended thirty-six festivals in sixteen countries. I did so because I needed to be reminded that there was beauty out there in the world, as I'd been watching the evening news a little too much. I wanted to feel a sense of wholeness with the world by tapping into people's collective effervescence. My more practical friends thought I was crazy or that I'd just become a party animal, but my intent was much deeper than that.

I made the pilgrimage to India's Maha Kumbh Mela, the largest collection of humans in history, to see tens of millions of ascetic Hindus show their sense of devotion to the sacred Ganges River. I discovered El Colacho, a four-centuries-old Pagan-Catholic annual festival, in a tiny Spanish village, that involves celebrating the triumph of good over evil by jumping over babies all day long. I was nearly gored by a bull in Pamplona, braved 30 degrees below zero (Fahrenheit) weather to marvel at the exquisite aesthetics of the Harbin International Ice and Snow Sculpture Festival in China, and studied the various rite-of-passage village celebrations that are a feature of life in Bali.

Again and again, whether it was witnessing ascetics or

aesthetics, I experienced the intangible, poignant value of community ritual. Not only did it make me feel part of a bigger whole, it made me feel holy.

Midlife: A Time for Wholeness

We are starved of this kind of communal joy in midlife. We miss a sense of discovery and play. Whether in a monastery or on the dance floor, midlife is the time to experience the feeling of being whole in the presence of others who are becoming whole as well.

We're not meant to be perfect in life, but we are meant to be whole. You may think you've shattered in midlife, but this is just because life is offering you (with the help of your family and friends) the opportunity to feel the sense of accomplishment to put yourself back together again piece by piece. Rest assured, you're not the only one doing this. You don't have to live a life of quiet desperation.

Most sporting matches get more interesting in their second half, and theatergoers sit on the edge of their seat during the last act of a play, when everything finally starts to make sense. Could it be that life, too, gets more interesting as one approaches its end?

Afterword: Why I Do This

*How many caterpillars does it take to spin a
chrysalis? One.
It's probably best to undergo our pathetic midlife
crisis alone. LOL.*

Midlife is not a crisis, it's a crossroads. But, unlike the
well-marked and well-tended road that we have taken up
to this point, midlife is bereft of road signs to help us navigate
the next stretch. I wish I'd seen the sign saying "Beware: Hair-
pin Turn Ahead" in my 40s or "Slow Down" in my 50s. More
than anything, midlife can feel like driving in the fog, so, even
if there are road signs, you don't see them. Most of us rely on
speed bumps, or life circumstances—like my cancer diagnosis—to slow us down so we can find our way.

Author Victoria Labalme writes,

In each of our lives at various points along the way, we
find ourselves in the Fog of Not Knowing—a period of
transition, when the path, the plan, or the project is not

yet clear.... This period "in between" — whether for minutes or for months — is to be respected and honored; it is fertile and full of promise. If you can meet this void without grasping for the most convenient way out, what you discover will be beyond your expectations and imagination.

I feel a deep commitment to this work of helping to rebrand midlife, partly due to my midlife friends who took their own lives and partly due to my own dark night of the soul. I wrote this book to help people clear the fog; to help them see midlife not as a source of dread or shame, but as the opportunity for reawakening.

I wrote it for people like Alison Franklin, whom I'd never met when she sent me an email that brought me to tears. She wrote that when she was a little girl, her mom playfully warned her, "Don't get old!" Her words legitimized a paradox Alison was already sensing: young is good; not young is bad. She vowed to defy her mother and Mother Nature. She would not get old.

For decades, she succeeded thanks to decent genes, dedication, and discipline. In her 30s and early 40s, she was in better shape than many in their 20s, and it showed. When she attended her twentieth college reunion in 2019, she silently awarded herself the superlative "Aged the Least" and felt triumphant. Alison was her own harshest critic but had trained for this milestone with injections, microdermabrasion, and twice-daily intensive workouts in a way that others clearly had not.

Alison continues, "Then the shit hit the fan. It felt like it happened overnight but was probably a gradual decline that I was too hardwired to take notice of." Her years of athleticism began to take their toll, leaving her with nagging injuries that limited her mobility and put her on the sidelines. "I couldn't sleep. I was paralyzed by dread, panic, and fatigue that my Type A personality and conscientiousness was no match for. I had always been acquainted with depression and anxiety but could no longer keep them at bay. I was not 'fine' anymore, and it rocked my world," she recalls.

Turns out Alison had gone through early menopause. Her thyroid stopped functioning and she developed other maladies that transformed her from, in her eyes, "high achiever to high-risk, deficient, suboptimal, low, slow and diminished." She was "an old woman trapped in a 45-year-old body."

Scarier than her physical ailments, though, was a profound fear that the best was behind her—and what if the "best" hadn't been all that good? What if she hadn't achieved everything that she was supposed to in the first act? Where was her consolation for hitting this impasse and hitting it early?

Alison continues, "I grapple with how to let go of my ego-driven perfectionism I've revolved my whole life around. I keep wondering, 'Is this it?' Yet my rigid, vapid values that no longer serve me are all I know. Without them, what would I have? Who would I be? What is my worth?"

Not long after her mom died of a rare bone marrow disorder, Alison started to reframe her relationship with midlife. In Alison's memories and photos, her mom remains ageless.

That's the irony: the biggest tragedy in her life is she didn't get the chance to grow old. Just when she lost her active lifestyle and the beauty that had once defined her, Alison found her mom's spirit, strength, and will to live—what she was really made of.

Alison finished the email by writing,

We don't get to choose between youth and aging. It's a disservice to think we do. I see that now. If we choose life, we will get older, we will have chin hairs and lose hearing and opt for practical footwear. I know there is only one choice but I can still be easily swayed into thinking there's another: whether it's a ponytail facelift, ice baths, curcumin. Chip, I appreciate you reminding me that growing and aging are the same thing.

Yes, we are aging and growing at the same time. And, ironically, it's our growing that helps us with our aging.

For me, midlife has been the best and worst of times. It's when I learned that getting older isn't about "growing up," it's about "growing into," especially when it comes to growing into our unique idiosyncrasies (and, trust me, I've got plenty). It's when I learned to find more comfort in the ambiguities of life. I've learned that when I am in a liminal state, I find all kinds of aspects of myself that were hidden in normal times. I feel honored being a midlife sherpa for others on their liminal journeys.

At each year's end, I rank my Daring Dozen reasons for

loving midlife just to see what's most resonating with me at that moment. My most recent ranking had chapter 7's topic (understanding my story) at the top and chapter 10's topic (time affluence) at the bottom, possibly because I was writing this book while running MEA and being an advocate for midlife in the world. I hope my list resonates with you, too. More than anything, I hope this book has helped make midlife aspirational for you.

My greatest reminder of why I do this work is hearing your stories. Please feel free to send them to me at stories@chipconley .com. On January 1, 2023, when I was in a deep funk about my time poverty, Alison's email came to me out of nowhere and was so perfectly timed. Thank you for sharing your vulnerability and courage with me and each other during this particular era of life. We're all better off for it.

Acknowledgments

I use the word *midwife* a lot in these pages, so let's give credit to these people whose midwifery skills made this a better book.

My agent Richard Pine has a finely attuned BS meter, so I was very encouraged when he told me this is a book whose time has come. He reconnected me with the insightful Talia Krohn, the editor of my last book, *Wisdom@Work: The Making of a Modern Elder*, who had moved to another publisher. I love working with her, as she's my "permissionary"—she gives me the permission to bare my soul on paper, but without going too far out, in my California lingo. Thanks to the rest of the Little, Brown Spark (Hachette) team, including Karina Leon, Juliana Horbachevsky, Betsy Uhrig, Sabrina Callahan, and Jessica Chun.

Bill Apablasa is the editor of my Wisdom Well daily blog and was a great collaborator on this book, which sprouted from my blog. Thanks to the following folks who read the manuscript and gave me thoughtful feedback: Jeff Hamaoui, Kari Cardinale, Leslie Bartlett, Gabriela Domicelj, Skylar Skikos (our fourth MEA partner), Barbara Vacarr, Eduardo Briceño, Marc Freedman, Barbara Waxman, Heather

McLeod Grant, Pat Whitty, Douglas Tsoi, Debra Amador DeLaRosa, and Vanda Marlow. (I'm sorry if I missed anyone.)

The foundation of many of the personal profiles in the book have come from the Wisdom Well blog's guest posts, and I want to acknowledge all the writers and say thank you. Many of these people are MEA graduates, so I want to say a huge thank-you to our full MEA team, especially those folks in Baja who've been with us for six years now. You create the conditions for our students to experience their transformative "Baja-ahas."

A big shout-out to Nicole Nichols and Gemma Korus for spreading the word on this book and MEA. They're creative, relentless, delightful, and full of integrity, which is impressive in the PR business.

My whirling dervish way of being is grounded by my family: my partner Oren Bronstein, Laura Spanjian, Susan Christian and our two sons, my parents, and my sisters, Anne and Cathy (Anne, I couldn't do all of this without you!), and my sweet Jamaican sister and housemate Cookie Kinkead.

Finally, the fertile ground of this book came from the soil of a few good souls who didn't make it through midlife. These friends in their 40s and early 50s—Chip, Brian, Arthur, Vince, and Vic—got stuck in their midlife chrysalis and couldn't find their way out of the goo. Gentlemen, you have been my inspiration in introducing this new road map for a life stage that is so deeply misunderstood.

Bibliography

WORKS MENTIONED

Brooks, Arthur C. *From Strength to Strength: Finding Success, Happiness, and Deep Purpose in the Second Half of Life.* New York: Portfolio, 2022.

Brooks, Arthur C. "No One Cares!" *The Atlantic* (New York). Nov. 11, 2021.

Brooks, David. *The Road to Character.* New York: Random House, 2016.

Grossman, Igor. "The Science of Wisdom." *The University of Chicago Center for Practical Wisdom* (Chicago). Oct. 15, 2020.

Hall, G. Stanley. *Adolescence.* New York: D. Appleton & Company, 1904.

Labalme, Victoria. *Risk Forward.* Carlsbad, CA: Hay House Business, 2021.

Manson, Mark. *The Subtle Art of Not Giving a Fuck: A Counterintuitive Approach to Living a Good Life.* New York: Harper, 2016.

Psaris, Jett. *Hidden Blessings: Midlife Crisis as a Spiritual Awakening.* Oakland, CA: Sacred River Press, 2017.

Rauch, Jonathan. "The Real Roots of Midlife Crisis." *The Atlantic* (New York). Dec. 15, 2014.

Rohr, Richard. *Falling Upward: A Spirituality for the Two Halves of Life*. San Francisco: Jossey-Bass, 2011.

Updike, John. *A Month of Sundays*. New York: Knopf Publishing Group, 1975.

Vanderbilt, Tom. *Beginners: The Joy and Transformative Power of Lifelong Learning*. New York: Knopf Publishing Group, 2021.

Vogler, Christopher. *Writer's Journey: Mythic Structure for Storytellers & Screenwriters*. Studio City, CA: Michael Wiese Productions, 1992.

Waldinger, Robert J., and Marc S. Schulz. *The Good Life: Lessons from the World's Longest Scientific Study of Happiness*. New York: Simon & Schuster, 2023.

Williams, Margery. *The Velveteen Rabbit*. London: George H. Doran Company, 1922.

Williams, Tennessee. "The Catastrophe of Success." *New York Times* (New York), Nov. 30, 1947.

SUGGESTED READING: CHIP'S TOP TEN MIDLIFE BOOKS

Angeles, Arrien. *The Second Half of Life: Opening the Eight Gates of Wisdom*. Boulder, CO: Sounds True, 2005.

Brizendine, Louann. *The Upgrade: How the Female Brain Gets Stronger and Better in Midlife and Beyond*. New York: Harmony Books, 2022.

Freedman, Marc. *How to Live Forever: The Enduring Power of Connecting the Generations*. New York: Public Affairs, 2019.

Hollis, James. *The Middle Passage: From Misery to Meaning in Midlife*. Toronto: Inner City Books, 1993.

Jackson, Mark. *Broken Dreams: An Intimate History of the Midlife Crisis*. London: Reaktion Books, 2021.

Lawrence-Lightfoot, Sara. *The Third Chapter: Passion, Risk, and Adventure in the 25 Years after 50*. New York: Sarah Crichton Books, 2009.

Levy, Becca. *Breaking the Age Code: How Your Beliefs about Aging Determine How Long and Well You Live*. New York: William Morrow & Company, 2022.

Rauch, Jonathan. *The Happiness Curve: Why Life Gets Better after 50*. New York: St. Martin's Press, 2018.

White, Elizabeth. *55, Underemployed, and Faking Normal: Your Guide to a Better Life*. New York: Simon & Schuster, 2019.

Zweig, Connie. *The Inner Work of Age: Shifting from Role to Soul*. Rochester, VT: Park Street Press, 2021.

Index

Calton, Joelle, 125–129
Campbell, Joseph, 112, 124
Carstensen, Laura, 29–30, 73–74
"Catastrophe of Success, The"
    essay (Williams), 149
"Cat's in the Cradle" song
    (Chapin), 165
Chapin, Harry, 165
Chesky, Brian, 11, 154–155
Chief professional network, 14
childhood self, learning from, 36
chrysalis metaphor, 7–8, 36–37
Clooney, George, 42
Cohn, Alisa, 46–47
collective effervescence, 71,
    200–202
communal joy, 200–202
comparing self with others, 63–64
compassion
    distilled compassion, 101
    emotional IQ and, 60
Conley, Chip
    core midlife, 11–12
    early midlife, 8–9
    experience with midlife
        midwife, 190–191
    exploring communal joy, 201
    Hero's Journey, 115–121
    midlife unraveling, 8–9
    "My Ten Commitments,"
        68–69
    near death experience, 10
    prostate cancer, 50–52
    role in Glide Memorial
        Church, 181–184

consumerism, 147
contentment, 57
"counterclockwise" experiment,
    31
Covey, Stephen, 92
Croce, Jim, 165
crystallized intelligence, 98

Daring Dozen list, 19–20
Dawn of Day, The (Nietzsche), 131
De Niro, Robert, 11
Dean, Teddi, 64
departure stage, Hero's Journey,
    112
disappointment
    frustration vs., 133
    managing, 132–134
distilled compassion, 101
Distinguished Careers Institute,
    14
Drucker, Peter, 106
Durkheim, Émile, 200
Dychtwald, Ken, 48

Edwards, Irene, 150–153
ego, 179–185
    overview, 179–180
    soul searching, 181–185
El Colacho festival, 201
emotional insurance, 74–77
emotional IQ (EQ), 58–62
    compassion, 60
    emotional fluency, 61
    environmental mastery, 61
    not taking things personally, 61

About the Author

Chip Conley has become a "CEO whisperer" as the mentor to countless young entrepreneurs, artists, politicians, and athletes. He has disrupted his favorite industry — hospitality — twice; first, when he was in his mid-20s, as one of the original American boutique hoteliers and then half a lifetime later as the "modern elder" to the Millennial founders of Airbnb. He was honored to be the "Most Innovative CEO in the Bay Area" by the *San Francisco Business Times*.

This is Chip's seventh book, and he's a *New York Times* bestselling author. Based upon his popular daily blog, Wisdom Well, he's considered to be the crossing guard at the dicey intersection of psychology and business. He's been a mainstage speaker at the TED conference multiple times, but he cares more about being a thoughtful leader than being a thought leader.

Chip's the cofounder and CEO of the Modern Elder Academy (MEA), the world's first "midlife wisdom school," where attendees learn how to reimagine and repurpose their lives with campuses in Baja California Sur (Mexico) and Santa Fe,

New Mexico. MEA has graduated more than 3,500 alums from 42 countries, and there are 26 regional chapters globally.

In the past few years, Chip's been on the boards of Burning Man, the Esalen Institute, Glide Memorial Church, Regeneration.org, CoGenerate.org, and the Stanford Center on Longevity. Chip holds a BA and MBA from Stanford University, and an honorary doctorate in psychology from Saybrook University. He has two sons, Eli and Ethan, as well as foster grandchildren and a foster great-grandchild. He lives near the MEA campus in Baja with his partner, Oren Bronstein.